THE HEART IN DIABETES

173. C.A. Nienaber and U.Sechtem (eds.): Imaging and Intervention in Cardiology. 1996
ISBN 0-7923-3649-6

174. G. Assmann (ed.): HDL Deficiency and Atherosclerosis. 1995   ISBN 0-7923-8888-7

175. N.M. van Hemel, F.H.M. Wittkampf and H. Ector (eds.): The Pacemaker Clinic of the 90's. Essentials in Brady-Pacing. 1995   ISBN 0-7923-3688-7

176. N. Wilke (ed.): Advanced Cardiovascular MRI of the Heart and Great Vessels. 1995
ISBN 0-7923-3702-4

177. M.LeWinter. H. Suga and M.W. Watkins (eds.): Cardiac Energetics: From Emax to Pressure-volume Area. 1995   ISBN 0-7923-3721-2

178. R.J. Siegel (ed.): Ultrasound Angioplasty. 1995   ISBN 0-7923-3722-0

179. D.M. Yellon and G.J. Gross (eds.): Myocardial Protection and the Katp Channel.
ISBN 0-7923-3791-3

180. A.V.G. Bruschke. J.H.C. Reiber. K.I. Lie and H.J.J. Wellens (eds.): Lipid Lowering Therapy and Progression of Coronary Atherosclerosis. 1996   ISBN 0-7923-3807-3

181. A.S.A. Abd-Elfattah and A.S. Wechsler (eds.): Purines and Myocardial Protection. 1995   ISBN 0-7923-3831-6

182. M. Morad, S. Ebashi, W. Trautwein and Y. Kurachi (eds.): Molecular Physiology and Pharmacology of Cardiac Ion Channels and Transporters. 1996
ISBN 0-7923-3913-4

183. A.M. Oto (ed.): Practice and Progress in Cardiac Pacing and Electrophysiology. 1996
ISBN 0-7923-3950-9

184. W.H. Birkenhager (ed.): Practical Management of Hypertension. Second Edition. 1996   ISBN 0-7923-3952-5

The Heart in Diabetes

edited by

John C. Chatham, John R. Forder

Department of Radiology, Division of NMR Research
Johns Hopkins University School of Medicine,
Baltimore MD 21205

and

John H. McNeill

Faculty of Pharmaceutical Sciences
University of British Columbia
2146 East Mall, Vancouver, British Columbia,
CANADA V6T 1W5

Distributors for North America:
Kluwer Academic Publishers
101 Philip Drive
Assinippi Park
Norwell, Massachusetts 02061 USA

Distributors for all other countries:
Kluwer Academic Publishers Group
Distribution Centre
Post Office Box 322
3300 AH Dordrecht, THE NETHERLANDS

Library of Congress Cataloging-in-Publication Data

A C.I.P. Catalogue record for this book is available
from the Library of Congress.

Printed on acid-free paper.

Printed in the United States of America

List of Contributors

Louis Arroyo, M.D.
The Department of Medicine
University of Medicine and
Dentistry of New Jersey
New Jersey Medical School
Newark, NJ 07103

John C. Chatham, D.Phil.
Department of Radiology
Division of NMR Research
Johns Hopkins University School of
Medicine
Baltimore, MD 21205

Vijayan Elimban, Ph.D.
Faculty of Medicine
Division of Cardiovascular Sciences
St. Boniface General Hospital Research
Centre, University of Manitoba
Winnipeg, Canada, R2H 2A6

Frederick S. Fein, M.D.
Department of Medicine
Albert Einstein College of Medicine
100 Morris Park Avenue
Bronx, NY 10461

David L. Geenen, Ph.D.
Montefiore Medical Center
Cardiology Division
111 East 210th St.
Bronx, NY 10467

Maren Laughlin, Ph.D.
Department of Surgery
Ross Hall 550
2300 Eye St
The George Washington University
Washington DC 20037

Alain Borczuk, M.D.
Department of Pathology
Albert Einstein College of Medicine
1300 Morris Park Avenue
Bronx, NY 10461

Naranjan S. Dhalla,Ph.D.,M.D.(Hon)
Faculty of Medicine
Division of Cardiovascular Sciences
St. Boniface General Hospital Research
Centre, University of Manitoba
Winnipeg, Canada, R2H 2A6

Stephen M. Factor, M.D.
Department of Pathology
Albert Einstein College of Medicine,
1300 Morris Park Avenue
Bronx, NY 10461

John R. Forder, Ph.D.
Department of Radiology
Division of NMR Research
Johns Hopkins University School of
Medicine
Baltimore, MD 21205

Leonard S. Golfman, Ph.D.
Faculty of Medicine
Division of Cardiovascular Sciences
St. Boniface General Hospital Research
Centre, University of Manitoba
Winnipeg, Canada, R2H 2A6

Gary D. Lopaschuk, Ph.D.
Cardiovascular Disease Research Group,
Departments of Pediatrics and
Pharmacology
The University of Alberta
Edmonton, Canada, T6G 2S2

Ashwani Malhotra, Ph.D.
Montefiore Medical Center
Cardiology Division
111 East 210th St.
Bronx, NY 10467

Timothy J. Regan, M.D.
The Department of Medicine
University of Medicine and
Dentistry of New Jersey
New Jersey Medical School
Newark, NJ 07103

Makilzhan Shanmugam, M.D.
The Department of Medicine
University of Medicine and
Dentistry of New Jersey
New Jersey Medical School
Newark, NJ 07103

Nobuakira Takeda, M.D.
Department of Internal Medicine
Aoto Hospital, Jikei University
Tokyo, Japan

John H. McNeill, Ph.D.
Faculty of Pharmaceutical Sciences,
University of British Columbia
2146 East Mall Vancouver
British Columbia
Canada, V6T 1Z3

Brian Rodrigues, Ph.D.
Faculty of Pharmaceutical Sciences,
University of British Columbia
2146 East Mall Vancouver
British Columbia
Canada, V6T 1Z3

Abbas Shehadeh, M.D.
The Department of Medicine
University of Medicine and
Dentistry of New Jersey
New Jersey Medical School
Newark, NJ 07103

Table of Contents

Preface

Diabetes is a major public health problem which is expected to affect 160 million people world wide by the year 2000. During the past 70 years the average life expectancy of diabetic patients has significantly increased; however, it is still substantially lower than the general population. Prior to the discovery of insulin the primary causes of death for people with diabetes were diabetic coma, infections and cardiovascular disease. The use of insulin has almost eliminated death from diabetic coma and dramatically decreased death from infections; consequently cardiovascular disease is now the leading cause of death in the diabetic population. Although cardiovascular disease remains the leading cause of death for the general population, diabetic patients have greatly increased risks of heart failure and coronary artery disease compared to non-diabetics. Furthermore, survival rates following acute myocardial infarction are markedly lower than the general population. Until recently the elevated risk of cardiovascular disease was presumed to be a direct consequence of the increased incidence of atherosclerosis in diabetes. Several decades of epidemiological and experimental research has suggested that there is a specific diabetes-induced cardiomyopathy that is independent of other risk factors for heart disease, such atherosclerosis and hypertension. Despite the impact of heart disease in limiting the quality and longevity of life for diabetic patients, there is no consensus as to the pathophysiologic alterations that are involved. Clearly an understanding of the effects of diabetes on the heart is an important step in the development of strategies to reduce the incidence of heart disease for diabetic patients, thus increasing their overall life-expectancy and quality of life.

In this book we bring together the different lines of evidence supportive of the idea of a diabetic cardiomyopathy. The first chapter provides an overview of the impact of cardiac dysfunction on the mortality and morbidity of the diabetic population in general, as well as a presentation of clinical aspects of heart disease in diabetes. This is followed by chapters concerned with the pathological and functional changes that occur in the heart as a result of diabetes and a description of the various therapeutic interventions that are available to reverse the effects of diabetes on the heart. Subsequent chapters focus on changes in protein synthesis, membrane function and intermediary metabolism that take place following the onset of diabetes. Since these alterations precede many of the functional and pathological changes, it may be that the processes responsible for the functional decline and tissue injury are initiated by diabetes-induced changes at the cellular and/or biochemical level.

CHAPTER 1

Clinical Manifestations of Diabetic Cardiomyopathy

Frederick S. Fein

The existence of a diabetic cardiomyopathy was first recognized by Rubler *et al.* in 1972, based on their study of four adult diabetic patients with both Kimmelstiel-Wilson disease and congestive heart failure [1]. None of their patients had evidence of valvular, congenital, hypertensive, or alcohol-related heart disease, nor of significant coronary atherosclerosis. The patients had diabetes for 5 to 20 years. Cardiomegaly was noted along with atrial and ventricular gallops and signs of pulmonary congestion. Left ventricular hypertrophy was present on EKG. Myocardial hypertrophy and fibrosis were noted on pathologic examination. In one patient, coronary arteriolar narrowing was present, owing to subendothelial fibrosis and accumulation of acid mucopolysaccharide (Fig. 1.1).

Epidemiology

In 1974, Kannel *et al.* described the influence of diabetes on the development of congestive heart failure as part of the Framingham study [2]. Diabetes was present or developed in 292 subjects; 4900 nondiabetic subjects were also studied. During an 18 year period, diabetic men had a relative risk of developing congestive heart failure 2.4 times that of nondiabetic subjects; the comparable value for diabetic women was 5.1 (Fig. 1.2). The age-adjusted incidences were 76 and 102 per 10,000 person years, or about 15% and 20% per person older than 20 years in men and women, respectively. In patients without prior coronary or rheumatic heart

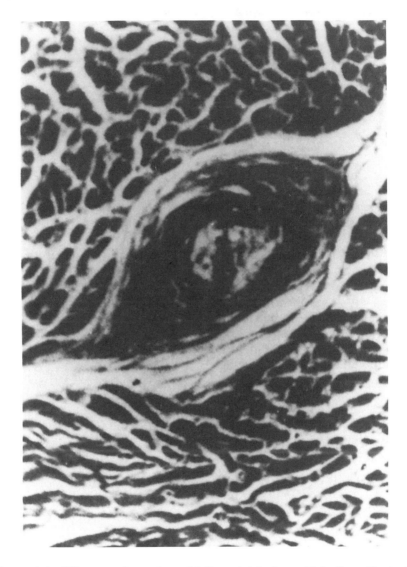

Figure 1.1: Microscopic section of left ventricle from diabetic patient with cardiomyopathy. A small intramural arteriole shows wall thickening owing to fibrosis and acid staining mucopolysaccharide material. (PAS; original magnification x 250.) (Rubler, S., *et al.*[1]; Reprinted with permission from American Journal of Cardiology: Vol.30, 1972, pgs595-602)

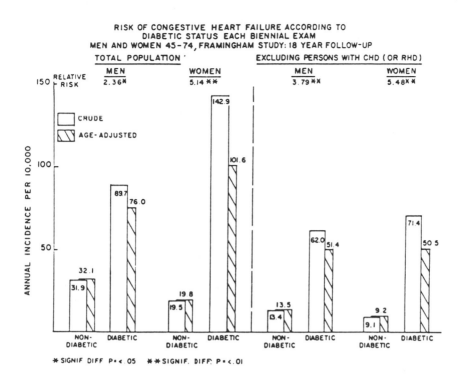

Figure 1.2: Risk of congestive heart failure according to diabetic status at each biennial examination. Data from Framingham study on men and women ages 45 to 74 years, with an 18-year follow-up. (CHD = congestive heart disease; and RHD = rheumatic heart disease.) (From Zoneraich, S: *Diabetes and the Heart.* 1978. Courtesy of Charles C. Thomas, Publisher, Springfield, IL.)

disease, a multivariate analysis demonstrated an increased incidence of congestive heart failure in diabetic patients, independent of age, systolic blood pressure, serum cholesterol, and Framingham relative weight. The subgroup of diabetic patients treated with insulin showed an increased risk of congestive failure, while patients treated with oral hypoglycemic agents or diet had no increased risk of congestive failure. Insufficient data were available relative to the influence of severity or duration of diabetes on the development of congestive failure. The diagnosis of coronary disease was made on clinical grounds; therefore, because diabetic patients may be more likely than nondiabetics to have silent myocardial ischemia, some subjects with diabetes and congestive heart failure might have been incorrectly assigned to the group without coronary heart disease [3-5]. Conversely, the incidence of myocardial dysfunction was probably underestimated, because only patients with clear signs and symptoms of congestive failure were included. Other epidemiologic data were provided by Hamby *et al.* in 1974 [6]. During a 6-year period, 73 patients with idiopathic cardiomyopathy were examined; 16 (22%) had diabetes. In contrast, in a group of 300 consecutive patients without cardiomyopathy (matched for age and sex), 33 were diabetic (11%). The frequency of diabetes in patients with congestive heart failure and in patients with cardiomyopathy, was significantly greater than anticipated. Almost all patients were more than 40 years old. The duration of diabetes in patients with congestive failure ranged from less than 1 year to 11 years. In contrast to the Framingham study, 15 of 16 diabetic patients with cardiomyopathy were treated with oral hypoglycemic agents or diet; only 1 patient was taking insulin. Thus, the relationship between the type of diabetes (and its therapy) and cardiomyopathy is uncertain.

Pathology

Cardiac histopathology has been described in diabetic patients with or without clinical evidence of congestive heart failure. Four patients with diabetic cardiomyopathy were studied by Rubler *et al.*, as described above [1]. Hamby *et al.* examined three such patients and also found evidence of myocardial hypertrophy [6]. Fibrosis was both perivascular and interstitial. In the small coronary arteries, endothelial and subendothelial proliferation with fibrosis was observed. The authors suggested that small-vessel disease could be responsible for the development of the cardiomyopathy.

In nine diabetic patients without significant coronary atherosclerosis (six of whom had evidence of congestive heart failure), postmortem examination by Regan *et al.* showed that heart weights were increased in some, suggesting the presence of ventricular hypertrophy [7]. Perivascular, interstitial, and replacement fibrosis with fragmentation or degeneration of myocytes was noted (Fig 1.3). Interstitial accumulation of periodic acid-Schiff (PAS)-positive diastase-resistant material was also

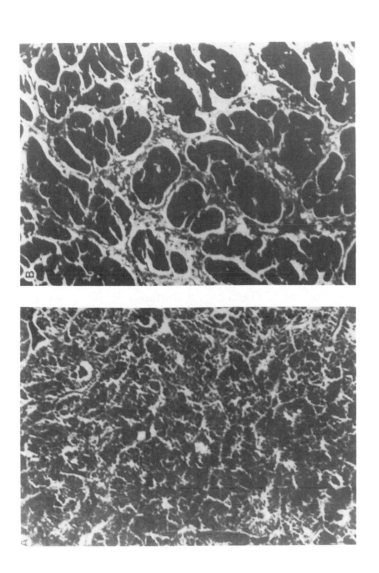

Figure 1.3: A, Microscopic section of left ventricle from nondiabetic patient with trichrome stain. B, Microscopic section of left ventricle from diabetic patient with trichrome stain. Deposits of connective tissue are diffusely scattered throughout the myocardium. (Original magnification, x 240.) (Reproduced from The Journal of Clinical Investigation,1977,Vol 60, pp885-889, by copyright permission of The Society for Clinical Investigation; Regan, T.J., et al.[7])

5

observed, presumably representing glycoprotein. Myocardial concentrations of triglycerides and cholesterol were diffusely increased. Pathologic changes within the small intramural coronary arteries were minimal or absent. In contrast to Hamby and co-workers [6], Regan *et al.* suggested that small-vessel lesions in diabetic patients may have little or no relation to the cardiac pathology [7].

A series of postmortem studies have been done in diabetic patients who did not necessarily have clinical signs of congestive heart failure. In 1960, Blumenthal *et al.* [8] described the intramural coronary arteries in 116 diabetic and 105 nondiabetic subjects. Large (160-500μm diameter), medium (70-150μm diameter), as well as small intramural vessels (20-60μm diameter) of diabetic patients more frequently exhibited endothelial proliferation with PAS-positive material interspersed between these cells than did vessels of nondiabetic subjects. These lesions were most frequent in medium-sized vessels, occurring in 66% of diabetic and only 28% of nondiabetic subjects.

Ledet found a higher incidence of PAS-positive vessels (20-60μm and 70-150μm diameter) in older diabetic patients (aged 50-70 years) compared to non-diabetics of a similar age [9]. However in contrast to Blumenthal *et al.* [8], there was no thickening of the vessel walls and no endothelial proliferation was observed. No correlation between the PAS-positive lesions and blood pressure was found. Another study by Ledet [10], of hearts from younger diabetic patients (aged 26-48 years) confirmed his earlier findings in older patients. In addition to the presence of PAS-positive vessels, perivascular fibrosis was present in these diabetic patients, and the number of medial cells was increased. In contrast capillaries were neither thicker nor more strongly PAS-positive in diabetic patients than non-diabetics; the capillary density was also similar in these two groups.

Zoneraich and Silverman [11] also described a high incidence of intramural coronary disease in diabetic patients, with pathologic findings similar to those of Blumenthal *et al.* [8]. In addition, myocardial fibrosis was frequently observed, particularly in patients with cardiomegaly. Crall and Roberts [12] described the coronary arteries in nine patients with juvenile onset diabetes and noted minor intimal fibrosis in the intramural arteries as well as

PAS staining of the media of some intramural arteries. In contrast, Sunni *et al.*, examining the intramyocardial vessels of diabetic and control subjects, found no histologic lesions that were specific for diabetes [13]. However, Tasca *et al.* found thickening of the intramural arteries from fibrosis and accumulation of neutral mucopolysaccharides; they also observed endothelial proliferation with focal protuberances which led to partial luminal narrowing [14].

Pathologic changes have also been documented in the capillaries of diabetic myocardium, in contrast to Ledet's findings [10]. For example, Silver *et al.* reported a threefold thickening of capillary basement membrane in diabetic patients, using tissue obtained at autopsy [15]. Fischer *et al.*, studying myocardial tissue obtained by biopsy during coronary bypass surgery, also observed capillary basement membrane thickening in diabetic patients [16], which was quantitatively greater in those with overt diabetes as compared to those with only glucose intolerance. An autopsy study by Factor and colleagues [17] using the technique of coronary perfusion with the silicone rubber compound Microfil, demonstrated capillary microaneurysms in three of six diabetic hearts (Fig. 1.4).

Studies of cardiac tissue obtained by biopsy, suggest a relationship between microvascular disease and diabetic cardiomyopathy. Right ventricular biopsy of diabetic patients without hypertension or coronary artery disease showed an increased myocyte diameter and increased degree of fibrosis; patients with positive exercise thallium scans had lower ejection fractions and tended to have a higher percent fibrosis [18]. The authors raised the possibility that abnormalities in the microcirculation may account for the abnormal thallium images in these patients. The results of another biopsy study showed arteriolar thickening, interstitial fibrosis, and basement membrane thickening in diabetic patients with an abnormal ejection fraction response to dynamic exercise and angiographically normal coronary arteries [19]. Thus a number of changes have been described in the microvasculature of the diabetic heart; however, it is still unknown whether they disturb coronary flow and contribute to alterations in myocardial structure and function.

The epidemiologic and clinical-pathologic studies discussed above emphasized the occurrence of cardiomyopathy in diabetic patients in the absence of hypertension. Factor *et al.* described the postmortem features of diabetic patients with severe congestive heart failure, all of whom were hypertensive [20]. Interstitial and

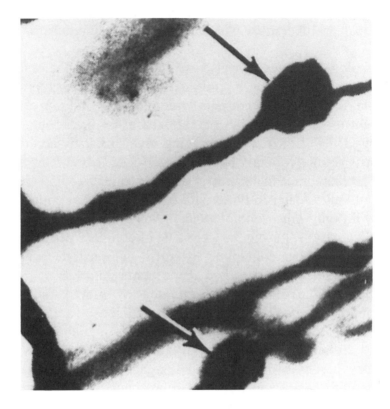

Figure 1.4: Cleared section of myocardium from diabetic patient perfused with Microfil. Two limbs of separate capillary loops are shown. Two saccular aneurysms are present, each of which measures more than three times the vessel diameter. (Transilluminated; original manifestation, x 900.) (Reprinted by permission of the New England Journal of Medicine (Vol 302, 384-388, 1980, Factor SM *et al.* [17]).

replacement fibrosis with myocytolytic necrosis were prominent in these patients' dilated and hypertrophied hearts. These changes were substantially more prominent than in patients with isolated diabetes or hypertension. The authors suggested that the combination of hypertension and diabetes may be particularly likely to lead to cardiac structural damage and heart failure. The concept that the two added stresses lead to increased pathologic changes is consistent with studies on the effects of hypertension on diabetic retinopathy and nephropathy [21-23]. Such findings take on added significance when the increased incidence of hypertension in diabetic patients is considered [24].

Cardiac catheterization

In 16 diabetic patients with a clinical cardiomyopathy, Hamby *et al.* found elevated left ventricular end diastolic pressure, whereas arterial blood pressure and systemic vascular resistance were normal [6]. Resting cardiac index was low in less than one half of patients and stroke volume index was normal in most. However, left ventricular end diastolic volume index was increased in almost all patients; consequently ejection fraction was markedly diminished. These findings are observed in congestive cardiomyopathy of any etiology. Left ventricular mass was uniformly increased. Coronary angiography revealed normal or at most minimally obstructed vessels. Regan *et al.* described the hemodynamic findings in four adult diabetic patients with heart failure and normal coronary angiograms [7]. Left ventricular end diastolic pressure was only modestly increased. Stroke volume index was low, whereas left ventricular end diastolic volume index was normal. The ratio of left ventricular end diastolic pressure to volume, a measure of wall stiffness, was increased. Ejection fraction was uniformly low and ventriculography revealed diffuse hypokinesis in three of four patients. These findings are consistent with a restrictive cardiomyopathy (contrasting with the findings of Hamby *et al.*[6]). Atrial pacing did not result in coronary sinus lactate production, suggesting that ischemia was not present.

The hemodynamic characteristics of diabetic patients who do not have clinical evidence of congestive heart failure have also been described. Independent of the duration of diabetes, diabetic men undergoing supine exercise had a lower cardiac output during exercise than did controls, without significant differences at rest, a result of a lower stroke volume [25]. In a later study, juvenile diabetics were examined shortly after diagnosis [26]. It was found that, although stroke volume during exercise was diminished in diabetic patients compared with controls, cardiac output was unchanged, due to a higher heart rate. A repeat study after 1 year of insulin therapy demonstrated reversal of these hemodynamic alterations. Regan *et al.* also evaluated diabetic patients without clinical evidence of heart failure and found an increased left ventricular end diastolic pressure but a diminished left ventricular end diastolic volume index, consistent with decreased compliance [7]. Stroke volume index was also low, but ejection fraction was normal, and the low stroke volume was attributed to diminished left ventricular filling. In conjunction with the hemodynamic studies in patients with clinically overt congestive heart failure, this study suggests that diastolic dysfunction may precede the development of systolic dysfunction in diabetic patients.

Noninvasive studies

The hemodynamic studies described earlier were primarily carried out in diabetic patients with clinical congestive heart failure. To learn more about the natural history of diabetic cardiomyopathy, noninvasive studies of the left ventricle have been carried out. Early work focused on measurements of systolic time intervals (STIs). Ahmed *et al.* [27] found a shorter left ventricular ejection time (LVET), an increased pre-ejection period (PEP) and an increased PEP/LVET ratio in asymptomatic diabetics who were not hypertensive and had no signs of nephropathy, retinopathy, or neuropathy. These findings were considered to reflect either decreased left ventricular contractility or decreased left ventricular filling due to diminished chamber distensibility. Seneviratne [28] also observed an increased PEP/LVET ratio in diabetics, but only in patients with evidence of retinopathy or nephropathy. However, Sykes and associates described somewhat different results [29]; PEP was shortened in a group of 19 diabetic patients prior to treatment with either diet or oral hypoglycemic agents. In diabetic patients requiring drug therapy, heart rate was increased and LVET was shortened before treatment. These abnormalities were reversed following a 3-month period of therapy. One interpretation of these results was that sympathetic tone was increased in untreated diabetics, resulting in an increased heart rate and shortening of STIs (even after correction for heart rate); with therapy, cardiac sympathetic activity presumably diminished,

10

leading to slowing of the heart rate and correction of the abnormal STIs.

Rubler and colleagues [30] noted normal baseline STIs in their population of diabetic patients, but observed that oral ethanol (in a dose producing no change in control STIs) caused an increase in PEP/LVET. Presumably ethanol made manifest the otherwise occult depression in myocardial contractility in the diabetic subjects. Shapiro *et al.* [31-33] found that PEP/LVET ratios were increased in untreated diabetic patients. In the less severely affected group, hypoglycemic therapy resulted in a decrease in this ratio. However, in a minority of patients where this ratio was markedly elevated there was no response after 4 months of treatment. Almost all patients with clinically apparent microvascular disease were confined to the group with persistently elevated PEP/LVET. Furthermore the subgroup of hypertensive diabetics also had a markedly increased PEP/LVET.

A large number of echocardiographic studies have been reported in diabetics. With respect to systolic function, several groups have observed decreased left ventricular fractional shortening, especially in diabetics with microvascular disease [28,31-37]. Takenaka *et al.* [35] found decreased fractional shortening in adult-onset diabetics only in those patients with left ventricular asynergy on echo; these patients had no clinical evidence of atherosclerotic coronary artery disease. In the Framingham study, Galderisi *et al.* [36] observed a slight decrease in fractional shortening in diabetic men. This abnormality was not independently related to diabetes but was accounted for by hypertension, obesity, and smoking. However, diabetes was an independent contributor to left ventricular mass and wall thickness. Vanninen *et al.* [37] studied newly diagnosed Type II diabetics and found decreased fractional shortening in female patients, which improved after 3 months of treatment (principally dietary management). Shapiro *et al.* [32] also found a high frequency of decreased fractional shortening in hypertensive diabetics. However, most investigators have not described systolic dysfunction in normotensive diabetics.

Abnormalities in diastolic dysfunction are more frequently observed in asymptomatic diabetics; however, using M-mode and Doppler echocardiography [30-33,38-43] Sanderson and colleagues carefully examined diastolic events and observed a variety of

11

alterations in left ventricular wall motion and mitral valve motion [38]. For example, 11 patients had a delayed mitral valve opening. Several subjects showed an altered relation between mitral valve opening and left ventricular wall motion; 3 patients showed substantial outward wall motion before mitral valve opening. Of interest, 19 of 23 patients had retinopathy, suggesting to the authors that the diastolic abnormalities may have been a result of myocardial small vessel disease. Uusitopa *et al.* [39] found prolonged isovolumetric relaxation and a lower peak diastolic filling rate in Type I and Type II diabetics, using M-mode echo. In this study there was no relationship between diastolic dysfunction and the duration of diabetes, the degree of metabolic control, blood pressure, or retinopathy.

Zarich *et al.* [40] observed a decrease in early atrial filling velocity and an increase in late filling velocity; the atrial contribution to stroke volume was also increased in diabetics. These abnormalities did not correlate with the duration of diabetes or the presence of microvascular complications. Sampson *et al.* [41] also found a decrease in the ratio of early to late filling velocity in Type I diabetics with proteinuria. In addition a slightly elevated blood pressure was observed in these patients, which correlated with both peak late (atrial) filling velocity and left ventricular mass. Riggs and Traisue observed an abnormal filling pattern in adolescent diabetics [42]. Vanninen *et al.* [37] found a decreased peak filling rate on Doppler study in men with newly diagnosed Type II diabetes, which improved after 3 months of treatment. Hiramatsu *et al.* [43] showed both prolonged isovolumetric relaxation and a decreased early to late (atrial) filling velocity ratio in Type II diabetics. This abnormality was exaggerated in patients with retinopathy, but only patients without retinopathy demonstrated a correction of the altered filling pattern after 1 month of insulin therapy. Recently, Raev [45] evaluated M-mode echocardiograms in 157 young asymptomatic Type I diabetics and found that diastolic dysfunction was twice as common as systolic dysfunction (27% and 12%, respectively). Diastolic dysfunction was observed an average of 8 years after the onset of diabetes whereas systolic dysfunction was observed an average of 18 years after the onset of diabetes. Microvascular complications were more severe in the presence of systolic dysfunction.

12

Consequently, Raev concluded that diastolic dysfunction occurs before systolic dysfunction in the development of diabetic cardiomyopathy.

Echocardiography has also been used to characterize abnormalities in myocardial tissue properties, using backscattering images. Perez *et al.* [44] observed altered acoustic myocardial properties in diabetics with normal systolic function, but subtle diastolic dysfunction, especially patients with neuropathy; this alteration may reflect increased myocardial collagen (See Chapter 3 for more details on the effect of diabetes on myocardial collagen).

Radionuclide ventriculography in diabetic patients has generally demonstrated normal resting ejection fraction but a lower ejection fraction in response to dynamic exercise. Some studies have shown a correlation between left ventricular systolic dysfunction and microvascular complications [19,46-51]. Mustonen *et al.* [52] found an abnormal ejection fraction response to dynamic exercise in Type I and Type II diabetics, independent of the degree of diabetic control, the presence of microangiopathy or autonomic neuropathy. In this study resting ejection fraction was normal in diabetic men but increased in diabetic women. However, Borow *et al.* [53] suggested that an abnormal ejection fraction response to exercise may not signify an abnormal contractile reserve in diabetics. They evaluated 20 Type I diabetics who were not hypertensive, some of whom had signs of retinopathy or autonomic neuropathy. One group had normal resting ejection fraction, which increased as expected with dynamic exercise. The other group had a higher than normal resting ejection fraction, which decreased (to the normal range) with exercise. The findings in the latter group were unrelated to autonomic dysfunction or to the presence of retinopathy. Furthermore, echocardiographic determination of a rate- and load-independent measure of contractility (before and after dobutamine infusion) showed normal contractility in both diabetic groups. The authors suggested that a specific diabetic cardiomyopathy did not exist. However, they did not evaluate diastolic function, and as has been discussed above, diastolic dysfunction is more consistently observed than systolic dysfunction.

In addition to changes in ejection fraction, radionuclide ventriculography has also demonstrated abnormal left ventricular

13

filling dynamics in diabetes [54,55]. Mustonen *et al.* [56] showed a decreased metaiodobenzyl-guanidine (MIBG) uptake in diabetics in association with diastolic dysfunction (using Doppler echocardiography). MIBG is a guanethidine analogue that participates in norepinephrine uptake by postganglionic sympathetic neurons. It was suggested that abnormal sympathetic innervation of the heart may contribute to diastolic dysfunction in diabetes.

The preceding discussion has focused on ventricular dysfunction in diabetics in the absence of coronary atherosclerosis; however, diabetic cardiomyopathy may also have a significant impact on the clinical manifestations of coronary artery disease. An early study by Dash *et al.* [57] argued against this conclusion. In this angiographic study diabetics had an increased prevalence of a cardiomyopathic syndrome defined by chronic heart failure, an ejection fraction below 0.48, and multiple widespread left ventricular wall motion abnormalities. However, the cause of this syndrome, specifically its relation to the extent of proximal coronary artery disease and the occurrence of multiple myocardial infarcts, was the same in diabetics and non-diabetics. They concluded that no additional factors such as a specific diabetic cardiomyopathy were necessary to account for the frequent cardiomyopathic syndrome in diabetics. A later angiographic study, by Wilson *et al.* [58] drew different conclusions. They observed a higher frequency of major stenosis in intermediate (but not proximal or distal) coronary artery segment in diabetic patients. However, the severity of coronary artery disease was not different in diabetics with or without signs of heart failure. Therefore, they concluded that it was necessary to invoke a diabetic microangiography or cardiomyopathy to account for the frequent occurrence of heart failure in diabetics with coronary disease. Interestingly, Wilson *et al.* [58] did not include ejection fraction in their definition of heart failure. Therefore, diastolic dysfunction may have been a greater factor in causing heart failure in these patients than in those of Dash *et al.*[57], all of whose patients had a subnormal ejection fraction.

Diabetic cardiomyopathy also influences the clinical response to acute myocardial infarction. Many reports have documented a higher frequency of congestive heart failure in diabetics in this setting, despite a similar or even smaller infarct size, determined enzymatically [59-61]. Stone *et al.* [62] evaluated ventricular function after myocardial infarction in diabetics and non-diabetics. Left ventricular ejection fraction was similar in both groups on admission. By 10 days after infarction, ejection fraction was lower in diabetics but the differences were small; mean values were 45.2% and 48.7% in diabetics and non diabetics, respectively. Despite this modest difference in ejection fraction, congestive heart failure developed much more frequently in diabetics during the early post infarction period (42.4% and 24.3% of diabetics and non-diabetics, respectively). At 3 months after infarction there were no differences in ejection fraction between the two groups. Nevertheless, the incidence of heart failure at 3 and 6 months after infarction was markedly increased in diabetics. The authors suggested that the frequent presence of heart failure in diabetics despite relatively preserved systolic function indicated that heart failure may be largely a consequence of diastolic dysfunction, a manifestation of diabetic cardiomyopathy.

Conclusions

A large body of evidence supports the concept of a diabetic cardiomyopathy, independent of coronary atherosclerosis. While the majority of asymptomatic diabetics have relatively preserved systolic function, diastolic dysfunction (reflecting increased interstitial connective tissue and/or slowed ventricular relaxation) is a more frequent event. In the presence of microvascular complications and/or coexistent hypertension, there may be progression to overt heart failure with features of either a congestive or restrictive cardiomyopathy. The control of hyper-glycemia and treatment of hypertension may be as critical to the prevention of diabetic cardiomyopathy as they are to prevention of retinopathy or nephropathy but clinical studies have not yet been carried out to evaluate the effects of these and other therapeutic approaches. The optimal antihypertensive agent is unknown, although the use of converting enzyme inhibitors in the treatment of diabetic cardiomyopathy is certainly reasonable, considering the utility of these drugs in the treatment of heart failure in general. Subclinical cardiomyopathy (especially diastolic dysfunction) probably has a major influence on the outcome of myocardial infarction in diabetics. The remaining chapters of this text will explore the pathophysiology and pathogenesis of diabetic cardiomyopathy.

References

1. Rubler S, Dlugash J, Yuceoglu YZ, Kumral T, Branwood AW and Grishman A. New type of cardiomyopathy associated with diabetic glomerulosclerosis. *Am. J. Cardiol.* **30**: 595-602, 1972.

2. Kannel WB, Hjortland M and Castelli WP. Role of diabetes in congestive heart failure. The Framingham Study. *Am. J. Cardiol.* **34**: 29-34, 1974.

3. Hume L, Oakley GD, Boulton AJ, Hardisty C and Ward JD. Asymptomatic myocardial ischemia in diabetes and its relationship to diabetic neuropathy: An exercise electro-cardiography study in middle-aged diabetic men. *Diabetes Care* **9**: 384-388, 1986.

4. Nesto RW, Phillips RT, Kett KG, Hill T, Perper E, Young E and Leland OS. Angina and exertional myocardial ischemia in diabetic and nondiabetic patients: assessment by exercise thallium scintigraphy. *Ann. Intern. Med.* **108**: 170-175, 1988.

5. Nesto RW, Watson FS, Kowalchuk GJ, Zarich SW, Hill T, Lewis SM and Lane SE. Silent myocardial ischemia and infarction in diabetics with peripheral vascular disease: assessment by dipyridamole thallium-201 scintigraphy. *Am. Heart. J.* **120**: 1073-1077, 1990.

6. Hamby RI, Zoneraich S and Sherman S. Diabetic cardiomyopathy. *JAMA* **229**: 1749-1754, 1974.

7. Regan TJ, Lyons MM, Ahmed SS, Levinson GE, Oldewurtel HA, Ahmad MR and Haider B. Evidence for cardiomyopathy in familial diabetes mellitus. *J. Clin. Invest.* **60**: 885-899, 1977.

8. Blumenthal HT, Alex M and Goldenberg S. A study of lesions of the intramural coronary branches in diabetes mellitus. *Arch. Pathol.* **70**: 27-42, 1960.

9. Ledet T. Histological and histochemical changes in the coronary arteries of old diabetic patients. *Diabetologia* 4: 268-272, 1968.

10. Ledet T. Diabetic cardiomyopathy: Quantitative histological studies of the heart from young juvenile diabetics. *Acta Pathol. Microbiol. Scand. (A)* **84**: 421-428, 1976.

11. Zoneraich S and Silverman G. Myocardial small vessel disease in diabetic patients. In: Zoneraich S., ed. *Diabetes and the Heart*. Springfield, IL: Charles C. Thomas, 3-18, 1978.

12. Crall FV and Roberts WC. The extramural and intramural coronary arteries in juvenile diabetes mellitus: analysis of nine necropsy patients aged 19 to 38 years with onset of diabetes before age 15 years. *Am. J. Med.* **64**: 221-230, 1978.

13. Sunni S, Bishop SP, Kent SP and Geer JC. Diabetic cardiomyopathy. A morphological study of intramyocardial arteries. *Arch. Pathol. Lab. Med.* **110**: 375-381, 1986.

14. Tasca C, Stefaneanu L and Vasilescu C. The myocardial microangiopathy in human and experimental diabetes mellitus. (A microscopic, ultrastructural, morphometric and computer-assisted symbolic-logic analysis). *Endocrinologie* **24**: 59-69, 1986.

15. Silver MD, Huckell VS and Lorber M. Basement membranes of small cardiac vessels in patients with diabetes and myxedema: Preliminary observations. *Pathology* **9**: 213-220, 1977.

16. Fischer VW, Barner HB and Leskiw L. Capillary basal laminar thickness in diabetic human myocardium. *Diabetes* **28**:713-719, 1979.

17. Factor SM, Okum EM and Minase T. Capillary microaneurysm in the human diabetic heart. *N. Engl. J. Med.* **302**: 384-388, 1980.

18. Genda A, Mizuno S, Nunoda S, Nakayama A, Igarishi Y, Sugihara M, Namura M, Takeda R, Bunko H and Hisada K. Clinical studies on diabetic myocardial disease using exercise testing with myocardial scintigraphy and endomyocardial biopsy. *Clin. Cardiol.* **9**: 375-382, 1986.

17

19. Fisher BM, Gillen G, Lindop GB, Dargie HJ and Frier BM. Cardiac function and coronary arteriography in asymptomatic type 1 (insulin-dependent) diabetic patients: evidence for a specific diabetic heart disease. *Diabetologia* **29**: 706-712, 1986.

20. Factor SM, Minase T and Sonnenblick EH. Clinical and morphological features of human hypertensive-diabetic cardiomyopathy. *Am. Heart J.* **790**: 446-459, 1980.

21. Knowler WC, Bennett PH and Ballintine EJ. Increased incidence of retinopathy in diabetes with elevated blood pressure. A six-year followup study in Pima Indians. *New Engl. J. Med.* **302**: 645-650.

22. Mogensen CE. Progression of nephropathy in long-term diabetics with proteinuria and effect of initial antihypertensive treatment. *Scan. J. Clin. Lab. Invest.* **36**: 383-388, 1977.

23. Mogensen CE. High blood pressure as a factor in the progression of diabetic nephropathy. *Acta Med. Scand. (Suppl)* **602**: 29-32, 1977.

24. Christlieb AR. Diabetes and hypertensive vascular disease: mechanisms and treatment. *Am. J. Cardiol.* **32**: 592-606, 1973.

25. Karlefors T. Hemodynamic studies in male diabetics. *Acta Med. Scand. (Suppl)* **49**: 45-80, 1966.

26. Carlstrom S and Karlefors T. Hemodynamic studies on newly diagnosed diabetics before and after adequate insulin treatment. *Br. Heart J.* **32**: 355-358, 1970.

27. Ahmed SS, Jafer GA, Narang RM and Regan TJ. Preclinical abnormality of left ventricular function in diabetes mellitus. *Am. Heart J.* **89**: 153-158, 1975.

28. Seneviratne BIB. Diabetic cardiomyopathy: The preclinical phase. *Br. Med. J.* **89**: 153-158, 1975.

29. Sykes CA, Wright AD, Malias JM and Pentecost BL. Changes in systolic time intervals during treatment of diabetes mellitus. *Br. Heart J.* **39**: 255-259, 1977.

30. Rubler S, Sajad MRM, Araoye MA and Holford FD. Noninvasive estimation of myocardial performance in patients

with diabetes: Effect of alcohol administration. *Diabetes* **27**: 127-134, 1978.

31. Shapiro LM, Leatherdale BA, Coyne ME, Fletcher RF and MacKinnon J. Prospective study of heart disease in untreated maturity onset diabetics. *Br. Heart J.* **44**: 342-348, 1980.

32. Shapiro LM, Howat AP and Calter MM. Left ventricular function in diabetes mellitus. I. Methodology and prevalence and spectrum of abnormalities. *Br. Heart J.* **45**: 122-128, 1981.

33. Shapiro LM, Leatherdale BA, Mackinnon J and Fletcher RF. Left ventricular function in diabetes mellitus. II. Relation between clinical features and left ventricular function. *Br. Heart J.* **45**: 129-132, 1981.

34. Friedman NE, Levitsky LL, Edidin DV, Vitullo DA, Lacina SJ and Chiemmongkoltip P. Echocardiographic evidence from impaired myocardial performance in children with type I diabetes mellitus. *Am. J. Med.* **73**: 846-850, 1982.

35. Takenaka K, Sakamoto T, Amano K, Oku J, Fujinami K, Murakami T, Toda I, Kawakubo K and Sugimoto T. Left ventricular filling determined by Doppler echocardiography in diabetes mellitus. *Am. J. Cardiol.* **61**: 1140-1143, 1988.

36. Golderisi M, Anderson KM, Wilson PWF and Levy D. Echocardiographic evidence for the existence of a distinct diabetic cardiomyopathy (The Framingham Study). *Am. J. Cardiol.* **68**: 85-89, 1991.

37. Vanninen E, Mustonen J, Vainio P, Lansimies E and Uusitupa M. Left ventricular function and dimensions in newly diagnosed non-insulin dependent diabetes mellitus. *Am. J. Cardiol.* **70**: 371-378, 1992.

38. Sanderson JE and Kohner E. Diabetic cardiomyopathy: An echocardiographic study of young diabetics. *Br. Med. J.* **1**: 404-407, 1978.

39. Uusitopa M, Mustonen J, Laakso M, Vaino P, Lansimies E, Talwar S and Pyorala K. Impairment of diastolic function in middle-aged Type 1 (insulin-dependent) and Type 2 (non-insulin-dependent) diabetic patients free of cardiovascular disease. *Diabetologia* **31**: 783-791, 1988.

40. Zarich SW, Arbuckle BE, Cohen LR, Roberts M and Nesto RW. Diastolic abnormalities in young asymptomatic diabetic patients assessed by pulsed Doppler echocardiography. *J. Am. Coll. Cardiol.* **12**: 114-120, 1988.

41. Sampson MJ, Chamber JB, Sprigings DC and Crury PL. Abnormal diastolic function in patients with type 1 diabetes and early nephropathy. *Br. Heart J.* **64**: 266-271, 1990.

42. Riggs TW and Traisue D. Doppler echocardiographic evaluation of left ventricular diastolic function in adolescents with diabetes mellitus. *Am. J. Cardiol.* **65**: 899-902, 1990.

43. Hiramatsu K, Ohara N, Shigematsu S, Aizawa T, Ishihara F, Niwa A, Yamada T, Naka M, Momose A and Yoshizawa K. Left ventricular filling abnormalities in non-insulin dependent diabetes mellitus and improvement by short-term glycemic control. *Am. J. Cardiol.* **70**: 1185-1189, 1992.

44. Perez JE, McGill JB, Santiago JV, Schechtman KB, Waggoner AD, Miller JG and Sobel, BE. Abnormal myocardial acoustic properties in diabetic patients and their correlation with the severity of disease. *J. Am. Coll. Cardiol.* **19**: 1154-1162, 1992.

45. Raev DC, Which left ventricular function is impaired earlier in the evolution of diabetic cardiomyopathy? An echocardiographic study of young Type I diabetic patients. *Diabetes Care* **17**: 633-639, 1994.

46. Vered A, Battler A, Segal P, Liverman D, Yerushalmi Y, Berezim M and Neufeld HN. Exercise-induced left ventricular dysfunction in young men with asymptomatic diabetes mellitus (diabetic cardiomyopathy). *Am. J. Cardiol.* **54**: 633-637, 1984.

47. Mildenberger RR, Bar-Schlomo B, Druck MN, Jablonsky G, March JE, Hilton JD, Kenshole AB, Forbath N and McLaughlin PR. Clinically unrecognized ventricular dysfunction in young diabetic patients. *J. Am. Coll. Cardiol.* **4**: 234-238, 1984.

48. Margonato A, Gerundini P, Vicedomini G, Gilardi MC, Pozza G and Fazio F. Abnormal cardiovascular response to exercise

in young asymptomatic diabetic patients with retinopathy. *Am. Heart. J.* **112**: 554-560, 1986.

49. Zola B, Kahn JK, Juni JE and Vinik AI. Abnormal cardiac function in diabetic patients with autonomic neuropathy in the absence of ischemic heart disease. *J. Clin. Endocrinol. Metab.* **63**: 208-214, 1986.

50. Harrower AD, McFarlane G, Paarekh P, Young K and Railton R. Cardiac function during stress testing in long-standing insulin-dependent diabetics. *Acta Diabetol. Lat.* **20**: 179-183, 1983.

51. Fisher BM, Gillen G, Ong-Tone L, Dargie HJ and Frier BM. Cardiac function and insulin-dependent diabetes: Radionuclide ventriculography in young diabetics. *Diabetic Med.* **2**: 251-256, 1985.

52. Mustonen JM, Uusitupa MIJ, Tahvanainen K, Talwar S, Laasko M, Lansimies E, Kuikka JT and Pyorala K. Impaired left ventricular systolic function during exercise in middle-aged insulin dependent and noninsulin-dependent diabetic subjects without clinically evident cardiovascular disease. *Am. J. Cardiol.* **6**: 1273-1279, 1988.

53. Borow KM, Jaspan JB, Williams KA, Neumann A, Wolinski-Walley P and Lang RM. Myocardial mechanics in young adult patients with diabetes mellitus: Effects of altered load, inotropic state and dynamic exercise. *J. Am. Coll. Cardiol.* **15**: 1508-1517, 1990.

54. Kahn JK, Zola B, Juni JE and Vinik AI. Radionuclide assessment of left ventricular diastolic filling in diabetes mellitus with and without cardiac autonomic neuropathy. *J. Am. Coll. Cardiol.* **7**: 1303-1309, 1986.

55. Ruddy TD, Shumak SL, Liu PP, Barnie A, Seawright J, McLaughlin PR and Zinman B. The relationship of cardiac diastolic dysfunction to concurrent hormonal and metabolic status in Type I diabetes mellitus. *J. Clin. Endocrinol. Metab.* **66**: 113-118, 1988.

56. Mustonen J, Martysaari, Kuikka J, Vanninen E, Vaino P, Lansimies E and Uusitupa M. Decreased myocardial ^{123}I-metaiodobenzyl-guanidine uptake is associated with disturbed

left ventricular diastolic filling in diabetes. *Am. Heart J.* **123**: 804-805, 1992.

57. Dash H, Johnson RA, Dinsmore RE, Francis CK and Harthorne JW. Cardiomyopathic syndrome due to coronary artery disease. II: Increased prevalence in patients with diabetes mellitus: a matched pair analysis. *Br. Heart J.* **39**: 740-747, 1977.

58. Wilson CS, Gau GT, Fulton RE and Davis GD. Coronary artery disease in diabetic and nondiabetic patients: a clinical and angiographic comparison. *Clin. Cardiol.* **6**: 440-446, 1983.

59. Partamian JO and Bradley RF. Acute myocardial infarction in 258 cases of diabetes. Immediate mortality and five-year survival. *N. Engl. J. Med.* **273**: 455-461, 1965.

60. Jaffe AS, Spadaro JJ, Schectman K, Roberts R, Geltman EM and Sobel BE. Increased congestive heart failure after myocardial infarction of modest extent in patients with diabetes mellitus. *Am. Heart J.* **108**: 31-37, 1984.

61. Gwilt DJ, Petri M, Lewis PW, Nattrass M and Pentecost BL. Myocardial infarct size and mortality in diabetic patients. *Br. Heart J.* **54**: 466-472, 1985.

62. Stone PH, Muller JE, Hartwall T, York BJ, Rutherford JD, Parker CB, Turi ZG, Strauss HW, Willerson JT, Robertson T, Braunwald E, Jaffe AS and the MILIS Study Group. The effect of diabetes mellitus on prognosis and serial left ventricular function after acute myocardial infarction: Contribution of both coronary disease and diastolic left ventricular dysfunction to the adverse prognosis. *J. Am. Coll. Cardiol.* **14**: 49-57, 1989.

CHAPTER 2

Pathologic Alterations of the Heart in Diabetes Mellitus

Alain Borczuk
Stephen M. Factor

The different clinical and pathologic manifestations of diabetes mellitus have fascinated those interested in this disease, regardless of their specific area of concentration. The severity of this systemic disease is reflected in the well known renal, retinal, neurologic and immune system consequences of diabetes. Improvements in the treatment of renal, metabolic, and infectious complications have increased the longevity of these patients, making heart disease an increasingly important contributor to the morbidity and mortality of diabetes.

There are several cardiovascular consequences of diabetes that impact on the heart to varying degrees. These include 1) accelerated atherosclerosis leading to coronary and cerebral artery disease; 2) systemic hypertension 3) microcirculatory injury leading to chronic multifocal myocyte damage and cardiomyopathy 4) neuropathy, specifically autonomic dysfunction 5) direct toxicity to the myocyte.

Coronary atherosclerosis

In the process of analyzing the damaging effects of diabetes on the vascular tree, one is on safe clinical, epidemiologic and pathologic grounds to begin with the epicardial coronary arteries.

These vessels, which are subject to atherosclerosis in non-diabetics, seem to be involved by atherosclerosis more frequently and more severely in diabetics, even when the data are corrected for hypertension, smoking, hyperlipidemia and obesity [1,2].

These data have come from a variety of sources, and appear to apply to type I and type II diabetics alike. The mortality rates from coronary heart disease (CHD) in type I diabetics begin to rise at age 30 and continue to increase in both men and women [3]. By age 55, the cumulative mortality was 35% in contrast to the significantly lower rates of 8% in non-diabetic men and 4% in non-diabetic women (Framingham Heart study). Mortality data for type II diabetics with coronary heart disease are no better, and CHD represents the most common cause of death in this population [4]. It is of interest that in addition to the Framingham data, studies of Israeli males from diverse countries of birth throughout Europe and North Africa [5] as well as studies of Japanese men and women [6] confirm an increased mortality from CHD in these populations. It is also of note that cardiovascular mortality has a greater impact on diabetic women (4.5 times greater than non-diabetics) than men (between 2 and 3 times greater) [1-3].

Mortality figures do not tell the entire story. The incidence [7,8] and severity [8,9] of coronary artery disease (CAD) at autopsy is increased in diabetics when compared with controls. The incidence has varied from two to eight fold greater in the diabetic population. In diabetics, clinical evidence of CHD correlated with the severity of CAD (degree of stenosis) [9], but not multivessel involvement or diffuse distribution [10]. Left main artery disease is generally more severe in diabetics than non-diabetics with CAD [9]. Type I diabetics show increased risk of CAD, with as many as 50% having either symptomatic or asymptomatic disease by age 55 [11]. When Crall and Roberts compared Type 1 diabetics with age matched controls (average age 29), the epicardial coronaries showed more than 75% occlusion in at least one vessel in diabetics; this was in contrast to age matched control cases that had minimal to no disease [12].

Cardiac imaging techniques have further supported these observations. Diabetics tend to have more extensive disease as defined by increased prevalence of multivessel and left anterior descending involvement [13,14]. Also found are higher left ventricular end diastolic pressures and increased incidence of left ventricular aneurysm. Neither increased distal nor diffuse disease has been documented. Although the incidence of CAD may correlate with "severity" of diabetes (as defined by insulin requirement) [15], no such correlation exists with the severity of the CAD (as defined by multivessel disease and extent of luminal narrowing) [7,8]. In addition, neither duration nor age of onset of disease is predictive of CAD [15].

Despite these varied sources of information confirming increased CAD in diabetics at an earlier age than non-diabetics, there is little morphologic support to explain these differences. In fact, there is no evidence that atherosclerotic plaque is any different in diabetics [16], with diabetic plaques having the expected intimal fibrosis, lipid deposition and calcification. There have been reports of a linear pattern of calcification within arterial tunica media that is radiologically detectable and associated with neuropathy and increased mortality [17,18]. Histologically, the main difference that has been repeatedly confirmed is the presence of periodic acid-Schiff (PAS)-positive material in vessel walls [12,19]. This material may represent basement membrane deposition in the intima and media, or deposition of advanced non-enzymatic glycosylation end-products in connective tissue [16]. The possibility that this material, at least in part, represents fibronectin has been suggested by immunohistochemical study of aortas [31]. In addition, smooth muscle cells in culture, when exposed to the serum of diabetics, make both fibronectin and basement membrane collagen [32]. These data suggest that at least part of the PAS positive material is type IV collagen and fibronectin. Finally, a non-atherosclerotic coronary artery disease in diabetics has been proposed, with the characteristic histologic changes including medial thinning [19]. It was also observed that in diabetics the tunica media outside plaques in proximal coronary arteries had increased amounts of connective tissue when compared to non-diabetic coronaries.

While morphology may have failed to yield major differences in diabetic macroangiopathy, biochemical and immunohistochemical study have shown some alterations in diabetes. An examination of aortas showed that all areas (both plaque and non-plaque) had increased medial but not intimal type IV collagen [20]. Type V collagen was not affected. A study of glycosaminoglycans (GAG) showed that diabetic atherosclerotic plaque had the same decreased ratio of heparin sulfate to dermatan sulfate as non-diabetic lesion [21]. What was remarkable, however, was that the non-atherosclerotic intima in diabetics showed the same altered ratio. If this altered ratio is a marker of ensuing atherosclerosis (since it is not present in non-diabetic, non-atherosclerotic intima), then diabetics may have an enhanced propensity to develop atherosclerosis. The alteration in GAG may be the direct result of the underlying insulin abnormality; however, endothelial injury, perhaps by lipid peroxides or hypertension, may also alter GAG synthesis.

Other studies have examined the effects of diabetes on hemostasis, including increased thrombin production, decreased fibrinolysis, increased platelet activity and circulating large platelets (for review, see 22,33). It is unclear whether hyper-coagulability causes acute arterial thrombotic events, occlusion of large vessel vasa vasorum, or exaggerated platelet response to endothelial injury; nevertheless the activation of platelets appears to play a role in accelerated atherogenesis in diabetes. Finally, the area of lipoprotein modification must be addressed, (for review, see 23-25). Glycated low density lipoproteins (LDL) appear to be particularly atherogenic as they are taken up by macrophages, creating foam cells. Its recognition by the LDL receptor is impaired [34]. Elevated very low density lipoproteins (VLDL) and triglycerides also contribute to atherosclerotic plaque. Further effects of glycation include possible immune complex formation with resultant stimulation of foam cells [35]. The cascade of lipid deposition, macrophage recruitment and phagocytic activity resulting in the fatty streak may be initiated by oxidized lipoproteins. Lipoprotein oxidation may in fact be increased by hyperglycemia, and direct endothelial damage and monocyte recruitment may be the result of increased oxidized LDL.

Although the exact mechanism of the vascular changes leading to accelerated atherosclerosis in diabetes is unknown, the result of increased CAD does appear to translate into an increased risk for acute myocardial infarction. In diabetics requiring insulin, the risk of myocardial infarction is 4 times greater than non-diabetics [26]. These differences are more marked for women than men, and the increased rate of myocardial infarction among non-diabetic males when compared to age matched females disappears in the diabetic population. Especially alarming, however, is the increased mortality after myocardial infarction amongst diabetics. Despite CCU care, mortality was two-fold greater for diabetics and this value worsened for those with poor glucose control [27]. This adverse outcome is observed in younger patients (less than age 65) and in women. Complications of myocardial infarction also appear to be more common, and these include atrioventricular conduction defects [28], reinfarction, congestive heart failure and late mortality [28,29]. Higher late mortality is also seen in diabetics who receive bypass grafts [30]. Interestingly, although congestive failure in diabetics is more common, infarcts do not appear to be more extensive [36]. It is possible that the effects of a systemic disease like diabetes on the overall health and survival of patients may account for these differences in outcome; it is also possible that associated illnesses such as hypertension may adversely affect prognosis. In addition, changes in the microcirculation resulting in myocardial damage observed in patients without significant coronary disease (to be discussed later in this chapter), may also occur in patients with CAD, enhancing complications and worsening their prognosis.

Hypertension

There is an increased prevalence of hypertension in diabetic patients over control subjects [37] with as many as 60% of diabetic patients affected. Interestingly women also suffer this complication more often than men of the same age [38]. Hypertension may be caused by changes in the arteriolar beds with widespread arteriolar hyalinization resulting in increased systemic vascular resistance; its end result can be devastating. Retinopathy and nephropathy are more common among hypertensive diabetics [39,40], and a lower rate of diabetic complications is observed in normotensive diabetics as well as in those treated with anti-hypertensive medications [41,42]. In cases where one kidney has a stenotic renal artery (thus protecting it from the effects of hypertension) only the unprotected kidney develops diabetic glomerulopathy [43]. The pathologic changes in the micro-

27

circulation that are worsened by a combination of diabetes and hypertension will be discussed in regards to cardiomyopathy.

Cardiomyopathy

Despite the higher incidence of coronary artery disease in diabetics, it is apparent that a certain number of diabetic patients develop congestive heart failure in the absence of significant coronary disease [44]. Over the past 15 years greater attention has been placed on further clarifying the nature of this cardiac dysfunction; the entity of diabetic cardiomyopathy has evolved and the important role of hypertension in the development of this cardiomyopathy has been recognized.

Despite the epidemiologic evidence for diabetic cardio-myopathy, little pathologic description of this entity existed. In 1980, Factor et al. [45], in attempting to better characterize diabetic cardiomyopathy, found that hypertension was a co-contributor in all the cases they identified. Further comparison of hypertensive-diabetic (H-D), hypertensive (H) , diabetic (D) and normal hearts from a larger group of patients led to the conclusion that hypertensive-diabetic hearts had more severe changes than the hypertensive or diabetic hearts alone [46]. In addition, hypertension alone had more severe effects than diabetes alone, though less than the cases with both diseases. The conclusion of these studies underscores the importance of hypertension in the development of diabetic cardiomyopathy, in that without co-existing hypertension, diabetic hearts are only mildly to moderately affected by cardiomyopathic changes.

The gross pathology of hypertensive-diabetic cardiomyopathy is characterized by left ventricular hypertrophy and increased heart weight [46]. An increase in right ventricular wall thickness has also been seen both in human and animal models of this disease [47]. This increase in weight as well as the relative right ventricular hypertrophy has been found to be greater in H-D hearts than in diabetic hearts alone. Extramural coronary disease was not present in these cases. Gross but non-segmental scarring was present to a greater extent in H-D hearts than in hypertensive or diabetic hearts. A firm ventricular wall with a waxy quality was also described. Finally, depressed, focal, discolored predominantly subendocardial

28

lesions were seen in H-D hearts and corresponded to areas of myocytolysis.

Histologically, the most notable features of these hearts was the presence of extensive interstitial fibrosis, around individual and groups of muscle cells, and replacement fibrosis [46]. The replacement fibrosis, defined by fibrosis that replaces myocytes causing focal scars, was examined at different stages of development and thought to be the end result of myocytolysis. PAS positive, diastase resistant material was present most commonly in H-D hearts, but was localized to areas of interstitial fibrosis and scarring. Areas of vascular sclerosis and perivascular fibrosis were present in H-D, H, D, and control hearts; PAS positive material was identified along with vascular sclerosis. Although the difference in numbers of affected vessels was similar in all groups, the extent of sclerosis and fibrosis was greatest in H-D and H hearts.

These light microscopic alterations lead to several theories as to the cause of cardiomyopathy and myocyte damage. These include intramural small vessel disease, abnormality of the microcirculation, accumulation of glycoproteins (especially non-enzymatic advanced glycosylation end products), direct myocyte toxicity or metabolic disturbances.

Investigations undertaken to confirm one or more of these possibilities revealed no correlation between small vessel sclerosis and fibrosis or myocytolysis. The pathogenesis of these myocardial changes was studied by using hypertensive-diabetic rats produced by renal artery clipping and streptozotocin treatment [48]. Combinations of myocytolysis and fibrosis were seen in these animals, similar to human hypertensive-diabetic cardiomyopathy. Furthermore, glycoprotein deposition as measured by PAS staining and small vessel changes did not correlate with the myocytolysis or the fibrosis [49].

Abnormality of the microcirculation that could not be detected by routine light microscopic examination became the leading hypothesis for the observed changes in myocardium. Post mortem human hearts were injected with silicone rubber solution and hardened *in situ* [50]. These studies demonstrated that some diabetic hearts contained the characteristics vascular changes of diabetic microangiopathy observed in the retina with microaneurysms in arterioles, capillaries, and venules. Also notable were tortuous and cork-screw vessels and vascular luminal narrowing with pre and post stenotic dilatation. These studies were then repeated in hypertensive-diabetic rats [51]. A similar injection of silicone rubber revealed microaneurysms, tortuosity and multiple foci of luminal narrowing, giving the vessel a beaded appearance. These changes were also seen, but to a lesser extent, in hypertensive or diabetic rats alone.

Examination of the affected vessels histologically failed to show any fixed anatomic lesions to explain the luminal narrowing. The vessels showed perivascular edema, fibrosis and inflammation. The possibility that vasospasm was responsible for these changes was entertained. Similar lesions in cardiomyopathic Syrian hamsters have been observed as a cause of multifocal necrosis and fibrosis [52]. Treatment with the calcium channel blocker verapamil prevented the histologic beaded appearance as well as myocardial necrosis [53]. In hypertensive-diabetic rats, treatment with diltiazem improved survival and showed trends towards decreased left ventricular fibrosis when compared to untreated rats [55].

Small vessel disease, as defined by myointimal thickening of coronary vessels (50-1000μm) leads to vascular compromise, ischemia and congestive heart failure in scleroderma and hypertension. Although seen in diabetics, no association between diabetes and small vessel disease is observed when myocardial biopsies are analyzed [54]. Sixty-one percent of biopsies, performed for diverse clinical indications, had small vessel disease, with hypertension as the only unifying diagnosis.

These pathologic alterations have physiologic consequences that have been measured by electrocardiogram, echocardiogram and stress testing. Untreated diabetics have resting tachycardia and shorter left ventricular ejection times than controls, and these parameters can be normalized with improved glucose control [56]. Small left ventricular end diastolic diameters, decreased stroke volume and thicker left ventricular walls have also been reported [57]. Inappropriate response of ejection fraction with exercise and elevated left ventricular diastolic pressures are also observed [58].

The effect of hypertension as a co-factor has also been seen in the clinical arena. Left ventricular function is worse in hypertensive diabetics than in hypertensives alone, and left ventricular diastolic dysfunction worsens with increasing systolic blood pressure [59]. Impaired left ventricular relaxation (decreased peak filling rate) and prolonged rapid filling period have been seen [60]. Systolic time intervals (pre-ejection period as compared to LV ejection time) are abnormal, possibly the result of decreased contractility or reduced preload due to decreased left ventricular compliance [61]. These findings have been seen in animal models of combined hypertension and diabetes, with prolonged contraction and relaxation, increased action potential duration, decreased resting potential, higher incidence of sudden death and circulatory congestion [62].

In summary, diabetic cardiomyopathy, especially with hypertension as an important co-factor, is characterized by interstitial and replacement fibrosis (non-specific histology for cardiomyopathy) in the absence of large vessel coronary disease or regional scarring combined with microcirculatory findings. Its existence has been supported by clinical testing in humans, physiological studies of rats, as well as pathologic studies of human and rat hearts.

Autonomic neuropathy

A systemic neuropathy is well described in diabetes mellitus, and its results on the gastrointestinal tract and on sensation are common clinical manifestation of this disease. An autonomic neuropathy also affects the heart. Loss of beat to beat variability and resting tachycardia is noted in diabetic electrocardiograms [63]. Decreased nerve velocities, improved by tight control, has been noted [64]. These effects on the parasympathetic system are followed by sympathetic dysfunction including hypotension with postural change. Sudden death is more common in patients with autonomic neuropathy [65]. Whether this is due to catecholamine hypersensitivity with resulting arrhythmia or if the frequency of painless myocardial infarction is higher is not known. Silent myocardial infarction has been described in diabetics as well in hypertensive and elderly patients [74], although it is not exclusive to this population.

31

Myocyte toxicity

Several derangements of intracellular myocyte metabolism have been described in animal models of diabetes, and some of these may influence cardiac function (for reviews, see 66,67; Chapters 7-10 also examine the effect of diabetes on cardiac metabolism). Dependence on lipid utilization caused by suppressed glucose intake results in higher triglycerides and free fatty acids in myocytes. Although ATP production remains adequate [67], the elevated intracellular byproducts of fatty acid oxidation may damage certain enzyme systems, including those of calcium transport in the sarcoplasmic reticulum [68]. This may result in altered contractility. Decreased calcium uptake [69], decreased calcium binding by the sarcolemma [70], decreased calcium intake by vesicles of the sarcoplasmic reticulum [71], and decreased myofibrillar Ca^{2+}-ATPase activity [72] have been shown in rat models, supporting the view that intracellular calcium defects may play a role in cardiac dysfunction. In addition, insensitivity to ß-adrenergic receptor stimulation has also been demonstrated [73]. (Chapters 3 and 6 discuss the role of altered calcium handling in the development of diabetes induced cardiac dysfunction). Protein synthesis is reduced in acute hyperglycemia. Insulin reverses many of these physiologic alterations. Although it is not clear how important any one of these elements is to diminished cardiac function in diabetes, the presence of abnormalities in calcium uptake and ß-adrenergic stimulation, correctable by insulin administration, is of interest in the overall understanding of myocardial dysfunction in diabetes.

Summary

The pathologic alterations in the heart in diabetes mellitus include coronary atherosclerosis leading to ischemic heart disease as well as microvascular injury resulting in multifocal myocytolysis, fibrosis and, eventually, cardiomyopathy. Hypertension, commonly seen in association with diabetes, may be an important co-contributor to vascular injury. Metabolic derangements may lead to direct myocyte toxicity, and cardiac dysfunction and metabolic effects may also contribute to accelerated atherosclerosis.

Ongoing study is needed to further understand the interaction of these simultaneous injuries with the goal of reversing their effects and decreasing cardiovascular morbidity and mortality.

References

1. Garcia MJ, McNamara PM, Gordon T and Kannel WB. Morbidity and mortality in diabetics in the Framingham population: Sixteen year follow-up study. *Diabetes* **23**: 105-111, 1974.

2. Kannel WB and McGee DL. Diabetes and cardiovascular disease: The Framingham study. *JAMA* **241**: 2035-2038, 1979.

3. Gordon T, Castelli WP, Hjortland MC, Kannel WB and Dawber, TR. Diabetes, blood lipids and the role of obesity in coronary heart disease risk for women in the Framingham study *Ann. Intern. Med.* **87**: 393-397, 1977.

4. Panzram G. Mortality and survival in type 2 (non-insulin dependent) diabetes mellitus. *Diabetologia* **30**: 123-131, 1987.

5. Herman JB, Medalie JH and Goldbourt V. Differences in cardiovascular morbidity and mortality between previously known and newly diagnosed adult diabetes. *Diabetologia* **13**: 229-24, 1977.

6. Sasaki A, Uehara M, Horiuchi N and Hasagawa K. A long term follow-up study of Japanese diabetic patients: Mortality and causes of death. *Diabetologia* **25**: 309-312, 1983.

7. Stearns S, Schlesinger MJ and Rudy A. Incidence and clinical significance of coronary artery disease in diabetes mellitus. *Arch. Intern. Med.* **80**: 463-469, 1947.

8. Vigorita VJ, Moore GW and Hutchins GM. Absence of correlation between coronary arterial atherosclerosis and severity or duration of diabetes mellitus of adult onset. *Am. J. Cardiol.* **46**: 535-541, 1980.

9. Waller BF, Palumbo PJ, Lie JT and Roberts WC. Status of the coronary arteries at autopsy in diabetes mellitus with onset after age 30. Analysis of 229 diabetic patients with and without clinical evidence of coronary heart disease and

comparison to 183 control subjects *Am. J. Med.* **69**: 498-505, 1980.

10. Dortimer AC, Shenoy PN, Sheroff RA, Leaman DM, Babb JD, Liedtke AJ and Zelis, R. Diffuse coronary artery disease in diabetic patients: Fact or fiction? *Circulation* **57**: 133-136, 1978.

11. Krolweski AS, Kosinsik EJ, Warram JH, Leland S, Busik EJ, Cader Asmal A, Rank LI, Christlieb AR, Bradley RF and Kahn GR. Magnitude and determinants of coronary artery disease in juvenile onset diabetes mellitus *Am. J. Cardiol.* **59**: 750-755, 1987.

12. Crall FV and Roberts WC. The extramural and intramural coronary arteries in juvenile diabetes. Analysis of nine necropsy patients aged 19 to 38 years with onset of diabetes before age 15 years. *Am. J. Med.* **64**: 221-230, 1978.

13. Schartz CI, Lesbre JP, Jarry G, Farchellone P, Kalisa A, Funck F and Simony J. Coronary artery disease in diabetes An angiographic study of 238 patients *Arch. Mal. Coeur* **76**: 872-877, 1983.

14. Vigorito C, Betocchi S, Bonzani G, Guidice P, Miceli D, Piscione F and Condorelli M. Severity of coronary artery disease in patients with diabetes mellitus Angiographic study of 34 diabetic patients and 120 non-diabetic patients. *Am. Heart J.* **100**: 782-786, 1980.

15. Lemp GF, Vander Zwaag R, Hughes JD, Maddeck V, Kroetz F, Ramanathan KB, Morris DM and Sullivan JM. Association between severity of diabetes mellitus and coronary arterial atherosclerosis. *Am. J. Cardiol.* **60**: 1015-1019, 1987.

16. Factor SM, Segal BH, and van Hoeven KH. Diabetes and coronary artery disease. *CAD* **3**: 4-10, 1992.

17. Edmonds ME, Morrison N, Laws JW, Watkins PJ. Medial arterial calcification and diabetic neuropathy. *Br. Med. J.* **284**: 928-935, 1982.

18. Everhart JE, Pettitt DJ, Knowler WC, Rose FA, and Bennett PH. Medial arterial calcification and its association with mortality and complications of diabetes *Diabetologia* **31**: 16-23, 1988.

19. Dibdahl H, and Ledet T. Diabetic macroangiopathy: quantitative histopathological studies of the extramural coronary arteries from type 2 (non-insulin dependent) diabetic patients. *Diabetologia* **30**: 882-886, 1987.

20. Rasmussen LM, and Ledet T. Aortic collagen alterations in human diabetes mellitus. Changes in basement membrane collagen content and the susceptibility of total collagen to cyanogen bromide solubilization *Diabetologia* **36**: 445-45, 1993.

21. Wasty F, Alavi MZ, and Moore S. Distribution of glycosaminoglycans in the intima of human aortas: changes in atherosclerosis and diabetes mellitus. *Diabetologia* **36**: 316-322, 1993.

22. Tchoepe D, Roesen P, Schwippert B, and Gries FA Platelets in diabetes. The role in the hemostatic regulation in atherosclerosis *Sem. Thromb. Hemost.* **19**: 122-128, 1993.

23. Ross R and Agius L. The process of atherogenesis- cellular and molecular interactions from experimental animal models to humans. *Diabetologia* **35**: S34-S 40, 1992.

24. Fineberg HN. Lipoprotein physiology in non-diabetic and diabetic states. Relationship to atherogenesis. *Diabetes Care* **14**: 839-855, 1991.

25. Chisolm GM, Irvin KC and Penn MS. Lipoprotein oxidation and lipoprotein induced cell injury in diabetes. *Diabetes* **41** (Suppl 2): 61-66, 1992.

26. Rytter L, Neck Nielsen H and Troelsen S. Diabetic patients and myocardial infarction. *Acta endocrinologica* **262**: S83-S87, 1984.

27. Harrower ADB and Clarke BF. Experience of coronary care in diabetics. *Br. Med. J.* **1**: 126- 131, 1976.

28. Czyzk A, Krolweski AS, Szablowska A and Kopczynski, J Clinical course of myocardial infarction among diabetic patients *Diabetes Care* **3**: 526-535, 1980.

29. Molstad P and Nustad M. Acute myocardial infarction in diabetic patients. *Acta Med. Scand.* **222**: 433-440, 1987.

30. Lawrie GM, Morris GC and Glasser DH. Influence of diabetes mellitus on the results of coronary artery bypass surgery *JAMA* **256**: 2967-2970, 1986.

31. Rasmussen LM and Heickendorff L. Accumulation of fibronectin in aortas from diabetic patients. A quantitative immunohistochemical and biochemical study. *Lab. Invest.* **61**: 440-446, 1989.

32. Rasmussen LM and Ledet T. Diabetic serum enhances synthesis of basement membrane like material in cultures of rabbit smooth muscle cells. *APMIS* **96**: 77-83, 1988.

33. Winocour P. Platelet abnormalities in diabetes mellitus.*Diabetes* **41**(Suppl 2): 26-31, 1992.

34. Lyons TJ. Lipoprotein glycation and its metabolic consequences. *Diabetes* **41**(Suppl 2): 67-73, 1992.

35. Virella MF and Virella G. Immune mechanisms of atherosclerosis in diabetes mellitus. *Diabetes* **41**(Suppl 2): 86-91, 1992.

36. Jaffe AS, Spadaro JJ, Schectman K, Roberts R, Geltman EM and Sobel BE. Increased congestive heart failure after myocardial infarction of modest extant in patients with diabetes mellitus. *Am. Heart. J.* **108**: 31-36, 1984.

37. Drury PL. Diabetes and arterial hypertension. *Diabetologia* **24**: 1-9, 1983.

38. Pell S and D'Alonzo CA. Some aspects of hypertension in diabetes mellitus. *JAMA* **202**: 104-107, 1967.

39. Knowler WC, Bennett PH and Ballintine EJ. Increased incidence of retinopathy in diabetics with elevated blood pressure A six year study in Pima Indians. *N. Engl. J. Med.* **302**: 645-650, 1980.

40. Krolewski AS, Canessa M, Warram JH, Laffel LMB, Christlieb R, Knowler WC and Rand LI. Predisposition to hypertension and susceptibility to renal disease in insulin dependent diabetes mellitus. *N. Engl. J. Med.* **318**: 140-145, 1988.

41. Christlieb AR, Kaldang A and D'Elia JA. Plasma renin activity and hypertension in diabetes mellitus. *Diabetes* **25**: 969-979, 1976.

42. Oakley WG, Pyke DA, Tattersall RB and Watkins PJ. Long term diabetes: a clinical study of 18 patients after 40 years. *Quart. J. Med.* **43**: 145-152, 1974.

43. Mauer SM, Steffes MW, Azar S, Sandberg SK and Brown DM. The effects of Goldblatt hypertension on development of the glomerular lesions of diabetes mellitus in the rat. *Diabetes* **27**: 738-746, 1978.

44. Kannel WB, Hjortland ML, and Castelli WP. Role of diabetes mellitus in congestive heart failure The Framingham study. *Am. J. Cardiol.* **34**: 29-38, 1974.

45. Factor SM, Minase T and Sonnenblick EH. Clinical and morphological features of human hypertensive-diabetic cardiomyopathy. *Am. Heart J.* **99**: 446-458, 1980.

46. Van Hoeven KH and Factor SM. A comparison of the pathological spectrum of hypertensive, diabetic, and hypertensive-diabetic heart disease. *Circulation* **82**: 848-855, 1990.

47. Fein FS, Cho S, Zola BE, Miller B and Factor SM. Cardiac pathology in the hypertensive diabetic rat. *Am. J. Path.* **134**: 1159-1166, 1989.

48. Factor SM, Bhan R, Minase T, Wolinsky H and Sonnenblick EH. Hypertensive-diabetic cardiomyopathy in the rat An experimental model of human disease. *Am. J. Path.* **102**: 217-228, 1981.

49. Factor SM. Intramural pathology in the diabetic heart. Interstitial and microvascular alterations. *Mount Sinai J. Med.* **49**: 208-214, 1982.

50. Factor SM, Okun EM and Minase T. Capillary microaneurysms in the human diabetic heart. *N. Engl. J. Med.* **302**: 384-388, 1980.

51. Factor SM, Minase T, Cho S, Fein F, Capasso JM and Sonnenblick EH. Coronary microvascular abnormalities in the hypertensive diabetic rat. A primary case of cardiomyopathy. *Am. J. Pathol.* **116**: 9-20, 1984.

52. Factor SM, Minase T, Cho S, Dominitz R and Sonnenblick EH. Microvascular spasm in the cardiomyopathic Syrian hamster. A preventable cause of focal myocardial necrosis. *Circulation* **66**: 342-354, 1982.

53. Factor SM, Cho S, Scheuer J, Sonnenblick EH and Malhotra A. Prevention of hereditary cardiomyopathy in the Syrian hamster with chronic verapamil therapy. *J. Am. Coll.·Cardiol.* **12**: 1599-1604, 1988.

54. Van Hoeven KH and Factor SM. Endomyocardial biopsy diagnosis of small vessel disease: A clinicopathological study. *Int. J. Cardiol.* **26**: 103-110, 1990.

55. Fein FS, Cho S, Malhotra A, Akella J, vanHoeven KH, Sonnenblick EH and Factor SM. Beneficial effects of diltiazem on the natural history of hypertensive diabetic cardiomyopathy in rats. *J. Am. Coll. Cardiol.* **18**: 1406-1417, 1991.

56. Fein FS. Diabetes and the heart. *Clin. Diab.* **9**: 83-91, 1991.

57. Shapiro LM. A prospective study of heart disease in diabetes mellitus. *Quart. J. Med.* **209**: 55-68, 1984.

58. D'Elia JA, Weinrauch LA, Healy RW, Libertino JA, Bradley RFand Leland OS. Myocardial dysfunction without coronary artery disease in diabetic renal failure. *Am. J. Cardiol.* **43**: 193-199, 1979.

59. Danielson R. Factors contributing to left ventricular dysfunction in long term type I diabetic subjects. *Acta Med. Scand.* **224**: 28-34, 1988.

60. Venco A, Granki A, Barzizza F and Finardi G. Echocardiographic features of hypertensive-diabetic heart muscle disease. *Cardiology* **74**: 249-256, 1987.

61. Sanderson JE, Brown DJ, Rivellese A and Volmer E. Diabetic cardiomyopathy: An echocardiographic study of young diabetics. *Br. Med. J.* **1**: 404-410, 1978.

62. Fein FS, Zola BE, Malhotra A, Cho S, Factor SM, Scheuer J and Sonnenblick EH. Hypertensive-diabetic cardiomyopathy in rats. *Am. J. Physiol.* **258**: H793-H805, 1990.

63. Page M and Watkins PJ. The heart in diabetes: Autonomic neuropathy and cardiopathy. *Clin. Endocrinol. Metab.* **6**: 377-390, 1977.

64. Cooper RS. Juvenile diabetes and the heart. *Ped. Clin. North Amer.* **31**: 653-663, 1988.

65. Ewing DH, Campbell IW and Clarke BF. The natural history of diabetic autonomic neuropathy. *Quart. J. Med.* **49**: 95-108, 1980.

66. Gotzsche O. Myocardial cell dysfunction in diabetes mellitus. A review of clinical and experimental studies. *Diabetes* **35**: 1158-1162, 1986.

67. Allison TB, Bruttig SP, Crass MF, Eliot RS, and Shipp JC. Reduced high energy phosphate levels in rat hearts: Effects of alloxan diabetes. *Am. J. Physiol.* **230**: 1744-1750, 1976.

68. Feuvray D, Idell Wenger JA and Neely JR Effect of ischemia on rat myocardial function and metabolism in diabetes. *Circ. Res.* **44**: 322-329, 1979.

69. Götzsche O. Myocardial calcium uptake in streptozotocin diabetic and control rats after dibutyryl cyclic AMP ß-adrenergic stimulation and calcium deprivation. *Acta Pharmacol. Toxicol.* **56**: 144-148, 1985.

70. Pierce GN, Kutryk MJB and Dhalla NSD. Alterations in calcium binding by a composition of the cardiac sarcolemmal membrane in chronic diabetes. *Proc. Natl. Acad. Sci. USA* **80**: 5412-5416, 1983.

71. Penpargkul S, Fein FS, Sonnenblick EH and Scheuer J. Depressed cardiac sarcoplasmic reticular function from diabetic rats. *J. Mol. Cell. Cardiol.* **13**: 303-309, 1981.

72. Pierce GN, Ganguly PK, Dzurba A and Dhalla NS. Modification of the function of cardiac subcellular organelles by insulin. *Adv. Myocardiol.* **6**: 113-125, 1985.

73. Atkins FL, Dowell RT, and Love S. ß-Adrenergic receptor adenylate cyclase activity and cardiac dysfunction in the diabetic rat. *J. Cardiovasc. Pharmacol.* **7**: 66-70, 1985.

74. Kannel WB and Abbott RD. Incidence and prognosis of unrecognized myocardial infarction: an update on the Framingham study. *N. Engl. J. Med.* **311**: 1144-1147, 1984.

CHAPTER 3

Alterations of Cardiac Function, Composition and Rhythm as a Consequence of Diabetes

Makilzhan Shanmugam
Louis Arroyo
Abbas Shehadeh
Timothy J. Regan

Introduction

The complex entity of diabetes mellitus has been a focus of cardiovascular studies in recent years. In terms of the heart a variety of investigations have defined diastolic as well as systolic mechanical abnormalities, electrophysiologic alterations, and multiple potential mechanisms. In this chapter we review the selected experimental data on the heart and relevant clinical information.

The relationship between diastolic dysfunction and collagen accumulation

Myocardial diastolic abnormalities have been described and attributed to an altered extracellular matrix. The myocardial interstitium has been the site of collagen accumulation in several species with diabetes, without evidence of hypertrophy [1,2]. Moreover the interstitium stains positively for periodic acid-Schiff (PAS) analogous to the renal mesangium [3].

The effects of chronic insulin use and tolbutamide were studied in male mongrel and canine dogs [1,4]. There was a significant rise in left ventricular end diastolic pressure with the infusion of saline with treated and untreated diabetic male mongrel dogs as compared to the normals. The tolbutamide treated and untreated diabetic animals showed a significant rise in left ventricular end diastolic pressure with the infusion of saline [4]. To examine the influence of diet on these myocardial alterations, a high or low lipid diet was fed to non-diabetic rhesus monkeys and a group with alloxan induced diabetes. Again, the diabetic group had a subnormal stroke work response compared to normals, as well as a significantly higher end diastolic pressure rise in response to normal saline [2].

In addition to animal studies diastolic dysfunction also has been observed in human subjects [5]. Although systolic dysfunction has been described with upright exercise, this was apparently secondary to altered preload conditions and was not seen in supine exercise [6]. As discussed in Chapter 1 diastolic dysfunction may precede the development of systolic dysfunction in diabetic patients. In general, systolic dysfunction is not normally observed in the subclinical state.

Collagen has been observed to accumulate in the myocardial interstitium of several species with diabetes without evidence of hypertrophy. Experiments in a canine model of diabetes have indicated that even in the mildly diabetic animal one can demonstrate a significant increase of interstitial collagen in the myocardium and diminished diastolic compliance without ventricular hypertrophy or evidence of ischemia [1,3]. This alteration has been observed in the monkey [2], rabbit [7], and some studies of rat [8], as well as human diabetics [9,10].

Observations in the hypertensive heart have revealed an apparent increase in collagen synthesis in the spontaneous hypertensive rat heart [11]. Ventricular hypertrophy was associated with enhanced and increased interstitial collagen volume [12]. This response was prevented by angiotensin converting enzyme (ACE) inhibition in a dose which did not affect hypertrophy, suggesting that the compliance abnormality was independent of the increased muscle mass. Recently, an increased ratio of Type I/III collagen was the specific abnormality observed in the same species, without an increase in total content [13]. This was normalized by chronic ACE inhibition. The reversal of the abnormality in these studies suggests that angiotensin II increases collagen synthesis, a finding observed in fibroblast cultures [12].

On the basis of solubility studies, collagen increments in diabetic myocardium appear related to diminished degradation rather than enhanced synthesis, since there was a decrease of soluble collagen and the total increments was solely represented by the insoluble fraction [2]. The relation of collagen solubility to synthesis is supported by data in a scleroderma mouse model in which an increased synthesis of this protein was associated with an increase of soluble collagen as well as the ratio of the soluble-to-insoluble fractions [14]. The persistent collagen increment in diabetes suggests the presence of irreversible advanced glycosylation end products.

It should be noted that in severe diabetes hydroxyproline accumulation may not occur over the long term, a finding consistent with impaired synthesis of cardiac protein during sustained ketoacidosis [15]. To assess the possible influence of exercise training on myocardial collagen, groups of exercised and non-exercised controls and alloxan induced diabetic dogs were formed. The concentrations of collagen in the left and right ventricles as well as septum were significantly increased in the non-exercised diabetics. Similar increments were not observed in the exercised diabetics in which the collagen concentrations approximated the normal control level [16].

Since growth hormone has been considered a potential basis for enhanced collagen synthesis, the relation of plasma levels of growth hormone to collagen accumulation was examined [17]. The levels of growth hormone in the basal state were similar in all four groups. After provocative stimulation with clonidine, which promotes release of the hormone from the pituitary, there was a progressive rise of growth hormone levels in the normals, that was similar in the sedentary and physically conditioned animals. The diabetic group exhibited a rise of plasma growth hormone that was not significantly higher in the non-exercised animals. This suggests that

43

collagen accumulation is not dependent on plasma growth hormone levels but the role of growth factors and cytokines is a fertile field for investigation.

Immunohistochemical studies of biopsies of myocardium using type specific anti-collagen antibodies were performed in 12 patients with IDDM and 6 non diabetic patients [18]. Exclusions included coronary artery disease, history of hypertension, chronic renal failure, or other endocrinological disorders. Substantial accumulations of collagen types I, III, IV in the myocardial interstitium were seen in both groups. The percentage of fibrosis in the sections stained with Mallory-Azan as well as type III collagen was significantly higher in the diabetic group than in the control group. The percentages of collagen types I and IV did not differ significantly between the two groups.

As a potential diagnostic tool, it has been suggested that collagen accumulation in the extracellular matrix of the heart is responsible for the abnormal acoustic properties of the myocardium in diabetic patients. Blunted cyclic variation of integrated backscatter and an increase in its phase delay may be an early sign of increased interstitial fibrosis in asymptomatic diabetics [19].

Development of systolic dysfunction during diabetes

Systolic dysfunction in experimental models of diabetes

Cardiac responses in experimentally induced diabetes are conditioned by the presence or absence of a chronic catabolic state. Systolic dysfunction has been shown principally in the latter model. Using the isolated perfused heart technique, Fein *et al.* [20] found systolic pressure as well as cardiac output to be less at higher filling pressures in chronically diabetic rats than in control animals. Analysis of the isolated ventricular papillary muscle revealed that the speed of contraction was diminished, as was the rate of relaxation. Because coronary blood flow was normal and there was no evidence of lactate production, ischemia did not appear to be operative. Concomitant biochemical abnormalities of the left ventricle related to systolic dysfunction included impaired Ca^{2+}-stimulated myosin ATPase activity and a switch in myosin isoenzyme from the normally predominant V_1 to enhanced V_3 levels [21]. Impaired calcium uptake by sarcolemma has been described [22]. Calcium binding and uptake by the isolated sarcoplasmic reticulum were also reduced, presumably contributing to slower myocardial relaxation [23]. An important observation was the normalization of these abnormalities when blood glucose was restored to control levels with long term insulin treatment.

A recent study in rats demonstrated that food restriction associated with weight loss can produce a diabetic type of myocardial dysfunction [24]. A close similarity between the effects of diabetes and food restriction on heart function, anoxic tolerance and response to the positive inotropic effect of calcium was present. These changes included increased contractility in atria, reduced contractility in ventricles, better anoxic tolerance, and a decreased positive inotropic effect of calcium in both atria and ventricles. The impaired function of the left ventricle was not significant until 4 weeks of diabetes or food restriction.

Cardiac abnormalities have been observed in two models of spontaneous diabetes. In the db/db diabetic mouse progressive damage to cardiac myocyte was observed which preceded the subsequent development of vascular lesions [25]. In this obese genetic model with insulin resistance [26], defective mitochondrial activity or altered lysosomal enzyme activity might be responsible for myocardial degeneration. The potential role of hypothyroidism in this model is not known. Moreover, the fluctuation of the glucose abnormality has raised a question as to the suitability of this model. Spontaneous diabetes in the BB/W rats resemble insulin dependent diabetes [27]. The hearts were studied at one, four and seven months after the onset of the disease and compared to age matched controls bred for resistance to diabetes. Calcium-activated myosin ATPase activity was significantly decreased after four months of diabetes with even greater abnormalities at seven months. These alterations were associated with reductions in the V_1 isomyosin content and an increase in the V_3 component. Since such alterations in the streptozotocin-diabetic rat were associated with depressed mechanical function, the authors inferred that contractility was impaired in this spontaneous model. Although thyroid levels were apparently normal, the presence of thyroiditis

45

in this model suggests a potential influence of this hormone on cardiac function in the diabetic state.

It is important to note that the altered cardiac characteristics in the rat model of diabetes are associated with non-pancreatic hormonal alterations. Both serum thyroxine (T_4) and triiodothyronine (T_3) have been found to be decreased in diabetic rats [28], similar to uncontrolled diabetes in humans [29]. Thyroid hormone has important influences on the myocardium. Sinus bradycardia, commonly present in the rat model, may be related to this apparent hormone deficiency. Serum T_3 and T_4 have been found to be depressed by three weeks after the onset of alloxan diabetes, when contractile function is reduced in the isolated perfused working heart. After treatment with insulin during the fourth week both thyroid hormone levels and cardiac abnormalities were restored to normal.

Treatment of diabetic animals with T_4 for five days prevented the decreased Ca^{2+}-activated myosin ATPase but did not prevent the changes of cardiac function, myosin isoenzyme or serum T_3 levels [28]. Use of pharmacologic doses of T_3 corrected the decrease in myosin ATPase and heart rate but only partially corrected the change in pressure development and myosin isoenzyme distribution. Cardiac function was restored to normal after increasing serum T_3 fourfold over a period of five days. In this model, the myocardial abnormalities may be largely secondary to the decline of thyroid function and diminished conversion of T_4 to T_3. Garber [28] has hypothesized that nuclear binding sites for T_3 are impaired in the heart and resistance to T_3 treatment necessitates larger doses to achieve normalization. Thus the relative roles of thyroid hormone and insulin require evaluation in the consideration of pathogenesis.

Systolic dysfunction in diabetic patients

The process of left ventricular hypertrophy has been more readily observed in humans than in animals. Female diabetics had greater subclinical abnormalities than male diabetics as described in the Framingham epidemiologic study [30]. Such abnormalities were also detected but to a lesser extent in females with glucose intolerance. M-mode echocardiography demonstrated increased left ventricular wall thickness, diastolic dimension, and left

46

ventricular mass. In diabetic men, fractional shortening was slightly reduced without an increase of left ventricular mass. Diastolic function was not evaluated. Glucose intolerance and diabetes were independent risk factors for electrocardiographic left ventricular hypertrophy from the original cohort of the Framingham study. Moreover, diabetic patients with left ventricular hypertrophy had a greater risk of cardiovascular events when compared to non-diabetics with left ventricular hypertrophy [31].

Another study of left ventricular systolic function utilized equilibrium radionuclide angiocardiography at rest, and during isometric and dynamic exercise in patients with type I and II diabetes without evidence of cardiovascular disease [32]. Abnormal left ventricular ejection fraction response to exercise was found in 42% of men with IDDM and NIDDM. In women, 71% of NIDDM and 44% of IDDM had an abnormal response. The validity of the finding of systolic dysfunction during exercise in asymptomatic diabetes has been questioned since load and rate-independent indices of contractility have revealed no abnormality [6]. These subclinical abnormalities support the concept of a chronic process involving the myocardium in diabetic patients.

The appearance of heart failure in diabetic patients in epidemiologic and hemodynamic analyses has been an important link in defining the course of the myocardial disease [9]. Hypertension and coronary disease as well as other etiologies of heart muscle disease were exclusion requirements. More than two thirds of the patients presenting with chest pain did not have significant coronary disease by angiography. There was no rise of plasma lactate levels in coronary venous blood during acute atrial pacing, supporting the view that ischemia was not present. End diastolic pressure was higher in diabetics than in age matched controls but with normal ejection fraction. The factors that promote progression of this cardiac dysfunction are largely unknown. However, the presence of even moderate obesity has been shown to be associated with an increased diastolic stiffness when compared to non-obese diabetics [33].

Progression to the first episode of congestive heart failure was attended by an interesting hemodynamic abnormality [9]. Although ejection fraction was reduced and filling pressure increased, end diastolic volume was minimally elevated. Thus, diminished diastolic compliance coexisted with abnormal systolic function.

Biochemical alterations related to systolic dysfunction

Depression of calcium uptake by the sarcoplasmic reticulum is associated with a rise of long chain acylcarnitine concentrations in this subcellular particle [23]. Elevated concentrations of circulating fatty acids may initiate a mechanism leading to defective calcium transport. Long chain fatty acyl CoA is also increased [22]. Alterations in calcium handling in the myocardium may also be due to alterations in membrane composition. In the rat with relatively severe diabetes the sarcolemma preparation isolated by ultracentrifugation has demonstrated a change in phospholipid content. Lysophosphatidyl content was increased while phosphatidylethanolamine was diminished [22]. Moreover, sarcolemma appeared to have an impaired capacity to bind calcium which paralleled a diminished sialic acid content in the cell membrane. Increases in cholesterol content of heart muscle have been consistently found in a variety of species, the rat [22], rabbit [7], dog [3], as well as humans [9]. The cholesterol increment appears to be somewhat equivalent over a wide range of diabetic severity appears to be closely related to the sarcolemmal fraction of the cell [22].

In moderate to severe diabetes, the accumulation of triglycerides in the heart [1] is associated with reduced total cardiac carnitine levels that appear to be due to lower serum carnitine levels [34]. Since carnitine is not synthesized in the heart, the myocardium relies on uptake from plasma for maintenance of intracellular levels. While transport of fatty acyl CoA across the mitochondrial membrane for oxidation is dependent upon the exchange of long chain acylcarnitine and free carnitine [34], reduction of the latter may contribute to lipid accumulation. Moreover hypoinsulinemia in diabetic animals may account for the increased levels of CoA in the heart [35], and further alter the CoA to carnitine ratio, a putative determinant of fatty acid oxidation. Hence esterification would be favored. See Chapter 10 for a more extended discussion on the effects of diabetes on fatty acid metabolism in the heart.

One of the more prominent contrasts between mild and severe diabetes is the presence of glycogen accumulation in the latter [36]. Glycolysis is inhibited at several sites in severe diabetes [37], and activation by an adrenergic agonist is anomalous. Severe diabetes decreases the ability of the ß-adrenergic agonist isoproterenol to induce changes in tissue content of cAMP and subsequently activate protein kinase [38,39]. (Chapters 8 and 9 discuss the effects of diabetes on myocardial glycogen and glucose metabolism in more detail.)

Alterations in protein metabolism would be expected to vary with the severity of the diabetic state although definitive information is lacking. In the intact rat made diabetic, the ribosomes present were somewhat less efficient in the synthesis of protein but the polysomes appeared to be maintained in the diabetic heart [15,40]. The ability to maintain peptide chain initiation was thought to be accounted for by the action of fatty acids in maintaining this process in heart muscle. The heart weight and RNA have been examined after aortic banding to evaluate the capacity of the diabetic heart to respond to an increase in afterload [41]. The hypertrophic response was similar to the controls after 10 days of diabetes in terms of heart weight. There was an increase in RNA content suggesting that protein synthesis was enhanced, but a role for diminished degradation was not excluded. (Alterations in protein synthesis as a result of diabetes are covered in Chapter 5.)

Altered electrical properties following diabetes

Altered electrical properties have been reported in the isolated superfused atria of rabbits with severe diabetes for three months. These were characterized by inhomogeneity of atrial conduction, atrioventricular conduction delay, slower sinus rate, and longer sinus node recovery time [42]. Action potential duration was prolonged in the basal state in studies of the rat papillary muscle following severe diabetes [43]. These cells reacted to ouabain or increased external calcium by a greater shortening of action potential duration than normals, thought to be due to alterations in the handling of intracellular calcium. The increased shortening of

49

action potential duration was enhanced in response to isoproterenol in a canine model of mild diabetes [16].

In diabetic rats there is a substantial increase in action potential duration which is secondary to a reduction in the magnitude and a slowing of the time course to recovery of the calcium-independent transient outward K^+-current [44]. At high rates, the prolongation of the action potential may limit diastolic filling and reduce stroke volume. The endocardial and epicardial gradient may be reduced or abolished secondary to the increased duration of the action potential. This may result in flattening or inversion of the T wave due to the pattern of ventricular depolarization. The prolongation of the QT interval in diabetics suggests that in the human myocardium as well there is an attenuation of the K^+-currents which repolarize the action potential [44].

Further observations in the diabetic rat have shown that the ventricular muscle of this species was more prone to develop delayed after-depolarizations and triggered activity [45]. This was observed under conditions presumed to produce myoplasmic calcium loading, after perfusion with ouabain or increased perfusate calcium. Alterations of ventricular vulnerability have also been reported in a canine model that exhibits glucose intolerance, with a small rise of glycosylated hemoglobin [16]. There was a significant reduction of the ventricular fibrillation threshold and a higher degree of spontaneous arrhythmias during acute occlusion of left anterior descending artery with a balloon catheter.

Although the autonomic nervous system has a crucial role in arrhythmogenesis, data on diabetic dysautonomia in animal models are rather scanty, but structural alterations of the sympathetic and parasympathetic nerve fibers have been described. Sympathetic nerves of the diabetic male Wistar rats showed significant neuronal and Schwann cell degeneration [46]. Whether this represents a basis for the impaired inactivation of norepinephrine by the uptake mechanism is not known. The normal release of tritiated acetylcholine, either basal or agonist stimulated, has suggested that post-ganglionic parasympathetic fibers remain intact during the first 3 months of experimental diabetes [47]. Treatment with insulin prevented or partially reversed some of the structural abnormalities in both sympathetic and parasympathetic nerve

50

fibers [48]. Similarly aldose reductase inhibitors improved sympathetic nerve function [49].

The incidence of sudden death has been observed to be high in diabetics versus non-diabetics [50,51]. However, the true incidence of arrhythmias in diabetic patients without evident ischemia is not known. Patients with autonomic neuropathy, more prevalent in type I diabetes, are considered to be are at particular risk. In humans, the circadian modulation of sympathovagal tone appears to be impaired in some patients with diabetes. The 24-hour power spectral analysis of R-R interval variability of 54 patients by EKG showed that diabetics with autonomic abnormalities had reduced low frequency bands when compared to normal subjects [52]. Moreover, the low frequency signals were greatly reduced nocturnally and during the first hours immediately after awakening, coinciding with the higher frequency of cardiovascular events. This reduction of vagal tone may result in impaired inactivation of norepinephrine by the uptake mechanism. In a recent study the 10 year survival of diabetics with symptomatic autonomic dysfunction was significantly lower than that of asymptomatic diabetics. However survival was as not closely related to R-R interval variability [53], used as a measure of autonomic dysfunction.

Subcellular changes related to altered electrical activity

A variety of tissue alterations have been observed in different diabetic models; in this section we focus on selected changes in a mild model of diabetes which may influence electrical or mechanical activity.

Alterations in intracellular cations -- Although reduced activity of cardiac Na^+-K^+ ATPase has been described in diabetes [54], a consistent change of myocardial potassium content in a canine model with mild diabetes and prolonged action potential duration has not been observed [1,7]. The normal concentration of cell potassium in the basal state is presumed to indicate that impaired activity of the Na^+-K^+ ATPase enzyme does not account for sodium accumulation in the diabetic model. A limited decline of Na^+-K^+ ATPase activity of approximately 20% may not affect cation transport [55]. In a more severe diabetic state with a decline of enzyme activity approximating this level, there was no decrease of potassium content in myocardium despite a significant increase of sodium content [56].

Two potential mechanisms for sodium accumulation are suggested. First a change in conformation of the ATPase may occur, so that there is an increase in high affinity sodium binding sites that face the intracellular compartment, resulting in high levels of sodium in the cell [57]. Alternatively, at an appropriate glucose concentration sodium may be less releasable from the cell membrane, a mechanism that may not affect the enzymatic site inhibited by digitalis. As a major regulator of sodium transport the sodium-proton antiport system must also be considered. Insulin is thought to reduce hydrogen ion concentration in the cell acutely, thus maintaining some degree of alkalinity [58]. Deficiency or impaired activity of this hormone may contribute to the accumulation of sodium, if there is an increased production of hydrogen ions in the cell. Under steady-state conditions, however, hydrogen ion concentration in the heart of diabetic animals has been shown to be normal [59].

Varied tissue calcium concentrations have been observed in diabetic models. Uptake of calcium has consistently been found to be impaired in sarcolemma [54] and diminished calcium activity has been observed in isolated cardiac cells of the diabetic rat [60]. Accumulation of cell sodium as a primary event would be expected to ameliorate the decrease of calcium by operation of the sodium-calcium exchange mechanism. However, an impaired function of the sodium-calcium exchange mechanism in the diabetic heart has been suggested, at least under conditions of ischemia with reflow [61].

Alterations in myocardial inositol content -- The reduction of inositol in cardiac tissue may affect phosphatidyl inositol composition and membrane function. Observations in the diabetic rat have indicated that ^{3}H-labeled inositol incorporation into phosphatidyl inositol, is significantly reduced [62]. Intervention with insulin was found to normalize the incorporation of inositol. A similar effect of hyperglycemia has been noted in experiments on aortic tissue; increased extracellular myoinositol selectively increased phosphatidyl inositol [63].

A recent report on the alloxan diabetic rabbit indicated no significant alteration in inositol content in whole heart; however, left ventricular concentrations were not provided [64]. Moreover, these studies were performed after 2 months in animals that were severely diabetic, in contrast to 12 months of a non-catabolic model. Accumulation of sorbitol has been described in several tissues in diabetes. However, the normal concentrations found here have been previously reported in the heart of relatively mild diabetics [65]. Thus, the inositol deficiency may well be independent of aldose reductase activity. The reduction of phosphatidyl inositol in cardiac membranes may contribute to the alteration of repolarization reported in the canine diabetics [16]. Whether sodium accumulation is related to these alterations remains to be determined. It is a reasonable to postulate that the lack of a concomitant potassium decrement may be related to an altered conformation of Na^+-K^+ ATPase so that high affinity binding sites release sodium less readily to the exterior of the cell [57].

Alterations in Norepinephrine Content -- The potential role of the sympathetic nervous system in this animal model of diabetes also needs to be considered. Enhanced release of norepinephrine (NE) from myocardium of diabetic animals without supplemental inositol was observed. In the mildly diabetic model, a secondary stimulation of the sympathetic system due to extracellular volume depletion appeared to be an unlikely mechanism for NE release since these animals maintained body weight and had normal extracellular volume in myocardium [66]. The significant reduction of NE release from myocardium in the treated group despite persistent hyperglycemia, may be related to correction of a sympathetic neural dysfunction due to an inositol deficit. Previous observations on the sympathetic nervous system have indicated depletion of myoinositol in the superior cervical ganglion [67], which may however, be limited to the early stages of the disease.

The decline of NE concentrations in the coronary venous effluent of the inositol treated diabetics does not appear to be related to hemodynamic factors. Heart rate, as the predominant factor affecting neurohormone concentrations in the coronary venous plasma [68], did not differ in the three groups, and was stable throughout the sampling period. A prior study of tissue NE in the rat after 6 weeks of diabetes has shown increased tissue concentrations as well as enhanced turnover in the left ventricle

[69]. Dietary myoinositol normalized these alterations. Although an excess of sorbitol was invoked as a mechanism for myoinositol depletion, the canine model with mild diabetes has not demonstrated accumulation of this polyol [66], which may however be related to its rapid turnover.

Increased NE concentration in arterial and coronary venous plasma was observed in the untreated diabetic animal. Central sympathetic outflow may be enhanced as judged by the reported increase in turnover of NE blockade [70]. Support for this view is provided by the increased activity of the enzymes related to catecholamine synthesis in the heart. Since these animals were severely hyperglycemic with plasma glucose higher than the threshold for renal excretion, the associated water loss may have been sufficient to reduce extracellular volume [71] and elicit secondary sympathetic stimulation.

The evaluation of NE and ^{3}H-NE levels in the coronary venous effluent of diabetics without the inositol supplement may be related to enhanced sympathetic neural activity or an impaired uptake mechanism. The significant increase of endogenous 3,4-dihydroxyphenylethylene glycol (DHPG), a metabolite of NE, is consistent with an increase of intraneuronal NE during stimulation. However, the lack of increase of ^{3}H-DHPG in the venous effluent during ^{3}H-NE infusion suggests that the NE uptake mechanism is impaired sufficiently to reduce the amount of ^{3}H-NE subject to oxidative deamination [72]. The catecholamine abnormalities were largely prevented by inositol feeding. Although changes of myocardial sodium and inositol were found in total tissue samples, the significant difference in NE metabolism suggests that cation and inositol content may have also been altered in the cardiac sympathetic nerves. In a freeze-fracture study, dietary myoinositol addition at the initiation of diabetes in the rat was found to prevent abnormalities of axonal plasma membrane in the dorsal sympathetic chain [73].

Ischemia and infarction

These syndromes occur in human diabetics, often associated with some degree of underlying myocardial dysfunction which may substantially modify outcome.

Animal data suggests that the underlying basis for ischemia, coronary atherosclerosis induced by diet, does not differ between diabetics and non-diabetics. When the rhesus monkey was made hypercholesterolemic, the presence of alloxan diabetes for 18 months did not appear to intensify the lipid streak lesion when compared to nondiabetics with equivalent levels of plasma cholesterol [2]. As an extension of that study, cynomolgus monkeys were fed a lipid diet which induced plaque lesions in the coronary arteries [74]. Physiologic and anatomic evidence suggested that the degree of atherosclerosis was no greater in the animals with induced diabetes. Coronary blood flow measured by the microsphere technique was similar in the basal state and an equivalent degree of ischemia was induced during vasodilation after adenosine infusion. Both groups exhibited similar degrees of subendocardial ischemia and depression of left ventricular function. In addition, the degree of intimal thickening and increase of arterial cholesterol and collagen content were comparable. Thus, at two stages in the development of atherosclerosis in hypercholesterolemic monkeys, there did not appear to be intensification of the process of the arterial disease by diabetes. This does not exclude an effect on the pathogenesis of complications such as ulceration or thrombosis that may take a longer time for development.

This observation is unexpected, in view of the putative abnormality of endothelium in some diabetic vascular beds [75]. However this may result in excess nitric oxide availability [76], which would tend to counter the increase of endothelial permeability during the development of atherosclerosis. The enhanced basal vasodilation associated with the relaxing factor may account for the relatively diminished coronary vasodilation after acetylcholine in diabetic patients compared to responses when basal tone is normal [77].

In the canine model of diabetes, coronary occlusion induced a significantly greater left ventricular filling pressure without a rise of volume, compared to non-diabetics [78]. The greater increase of myocardial stiffness was associated with a larger decline of systolic function. Coronary blood flow reduction and the size of the ischemic area were comparable.

A clinical counterpart to this finding has been observed in diabetics undergoing an initial acute infarction without other risk factors [79]. There was a seven fold increase in 30 day mortality compared to non-diabetics, largely due to cardiac failure. This outcome appears to be substantially improved by the use of new therapeutic modalities [80]. It is noteworthy that alterations of intramural vessels have been considered to contribute to reduced myocardial perfusion in diabetes. However a post mortem study, which examined vessels of varied size over a wide area of myocardium, found no significant difference in luminal area compared to non-diabetic controls [81]. This finding, in contrast to prior reports, was attributed to the coronary perfusion-fixation technique used to approximate the *in vivo* dimensions of the vascular lumen.

The basis for the exaggerated left ventricular dysfunction in diabetics is presumably multifactorial. Pre-existent enhanced diastolic stiffness presumably contributes to the development of heart failure after infarction. This process, related to interstitial fibrosis, would limit the compensatory responses of the non-ischemic myocardium. The ischemic myocytes at the margin of the infarct may have less capacity for recovery than in nondiabetics. In addition abnormalities of substrate metabolism as well as altered systemic and local neurohormonal mechanisms presumably contribute to the clinical outcome.

Summary

Several species with diabetes (dog, monkey, rabbits, humans) have shown an increase in interstitial collagen and diminished left ventricular diastolic compliance that were both refractory to insulin therapy. On the basis of solubility studies, collagen increments in diabetic myocardium appear related to diminished degradation rather than enhanced synthesis, since there was a decrease of soluble collagen and a rise of the insoluble fraction, presumably related to enhanced cross-linkage. The latter was associated with irreversible advanced glycosylation end products. This process is retarded by the early introduction of an exercise program.

The observed sodium accumulation without potassium loss in the cell may be secondary to a change in the conformation of ATPase or an alteration in the sodium hydrogen antiport system. However an impaired potassium current has been associated with a prolonged repolarization time which may facilitate re-entry arrhythmias, particularly in the presence of interstitial fibrosis. Calcium uptake has consistently been found to be impaired in sarcolemma. Isolated cardiac cells of diabetic rats have shown diminished calcium activity. Sodium-calcium exchange may be impaired, at least under conditions of ischemia with reperfusion.

A reduction of inositol in cardiac tissue has been associated with a reduction of phosphatidyl inositol and membrane function. Insulin corrects this abnormality. The altered membrane composition may have an effect on sodium accumulation that has yet to be defined.

The left ventricular myocardium of the diabetic dog has demonstrated a significant overflow of norepinephrine, due to an impaired re-uptake mechanism. Chronic feeding of inositol corrected this sympathetic abnormality. A functional correlate was observed in terms of rhythmicity. The diabetic dog exhibits a significant reduction of the ventricular fibrillation threshold, paralleled by an increased incidence of spontaneous fibrillation during acute regional ischemia. In the canine model fed inositol from the onset of diabetes the fibrillation threshold remained normal.

References

1. Regan TJ, Wu CF, Yeh CK, Oldewurtel HA and Haider B. Myocardial composition and function in diabetes: the effects of chronic insulin use. *Circ. Res.* **49**: 1268-1277, 1981.

2. Haider B, Yeh CK and Thomas G. Influence of diabetes on the myocardium and coronary arteries of rhesus monkey fed an atherogenic diet. *Circ. Res.* **49**: 1278-1288.1981.

3. Regan TJ, Ettinger PO, Kahn MI, Jesrani MU, Lyons MM, Oldewurtel HA, and Weber M. Altered Myocardial Function and Metabolism in Chronic Diabetes Mellitus without Ischemia in Dogs. *Circ. Res.* **35**: 222-237, 1974.

4. Wu CF, Haider B, Ahmed S, Oldewurted HA, Lyons MM and Regan TJ. The effects of Tolbutamide on the myocardium in experimental diabetes. *Circulation* **55**: 200-205.1977.

5. Shehadeh A and Regan TJ. Cardiac Consequences of Diabetes. *Clin.Cardiol.* **18**: 301-305,1995.

6. Borow KM, Jaspan JB, Williams KA, Newmann A, Wolinski-Walley P and Lang RM. Myocardial mechanics in young adult patients with diabetes mellitus: Effects of altered load, ionotropic states and dynamic exercise. *J. Am. Coll. Cardiol* **15**: 1508-1517

7. Bhimji S, Godin DV and McNeill JH. Biochemical and Functional Changes in Hearts from Rabbits with Diabetes. *Diabetologia* **18**: 452-457, 1985.

8. Baandrup V, Ledet T and Raxch R. Experimental diabetic cardiopathy preventable by insulin treatment. *Lab. Invest.* **45**: 169-173, 1981.

9. Regan, TJ, Lyons MM, Ahmed SS, Levinson GE, Oldewurtel HA, Ahmad MR and Haider B. Evidence for cardiomyopathy in Familial Diabetes Mellitus. *J. Clin. Invest.* **60**: 885-899, 1977.

10. Genda A, Mizuno S, Nunoda S, Nakayama A, Igarashi Y, Sugihara N, Namura M, Takeda R, Bunko H and Hisada K. Clinical Studies on Diabetes using exercise testing with myocardial scintigraphy and endomyocardial biopsy. *Clin Cardiol.* **9**: 375-382, 1986.

11. Van Hoeven KH and Factor SM. A comparison of the pathological spectrum of hypertensive, diabetic and hypertensive-diabetic heart disease. *Circulation* **82**: 848-855, 1990.

12. Brilla CG, Janicki JS and Weber KT. Impaired diastolic function and coronary reserve in genetic hypertension. *Circ. Res.* **69**: 107-115, 1991

13. Sen S and Mukherjee D. Alteration of cardiac collagen phenotypes in hypertensive hypertrophy: Role of blood pressure. *J. Mol. Cell. Cardiol.* **25**: 185-196, 1993.

14. Chapman D and Eghbali M. Expression of fibrillar types I and III and basement membrane collagen type IV genes in Myocardium of tight skin mouse. *Cardiovasc. Res.* **24**: 578-583, 1990.

15. Pain VM and Garlick RJ. Effects of streptozotocin diabetes and insulin treatment on the rate of protein synthesis in tissues of the rat in vivo. *J. Biol. Chem.* **279**: 4510-4514, 1974.

16. Bakth S, Arena J, Lee W, Torres R, Haider B and Patel BC. Arrhythmia susceptibility and myocardial composition in diabetes. Influence of physical conditioning. *J. Clin. Invest.* 77: 382-395, 1986.

17. Regan TJ, Alszuler N, Eddy C and Bakth S. Relation of growth hormone and myocardial collagen accumulation in experimental diabetes. *J. Lab. Clin. Med.* **110**: 274-278, 1987.

18. Shimizu M, Umeda K, Sugihara N, Yoshio H,Ino H, Takeda R, Okada Y and Nakanishi I. Collagen remodeling in myocardia of patients with diabetes. *J. Clin. Pathology.* **46**: 32-36, 1993.

19. Perez JE, McGill JB, Santiago J. Schechtmann KB, Wagner AD, Miller JG and Sobel BE. Abnormal myocardial acoustic properties in diabetic patients and their correlation with the severity of the disease. *J. Am. Coll. Cardiol.* **19**: 1154-1162, 1992.

20. Fein FS, Kornstein LB, Strobeck JE, Capasso JM and Sonneblick EH. Altered myocardial mechanics in diabetic patients and their correlation with the severity of the disease. *J. Am. Coll. Cardiol.* **47**: 922-933, 1981.

21. Malhotra A, Penpargkul S, Fein F, Sonnenblick EH and Scheuer J. The effect of streptozocin-induced diabetes in rats on cardiac contractile proteins. *Circ. Res.* **49**: 1243-1250, 1981

22. Pierce GN, Kutryk MJB and Dhalla NS. Alterations in calcium binding and composition of cardiac sarcolemmal membrane in chronic diabetes. *Proc Natl Acad Sci USA* **80**: 5412-5416, 1983.

23. Lopaschuk GD, Tahiliani AG, Vadlamudi RVSV, Katz S and McNeill JH. Cardiac sarcoplasmic reticulum function in insulin or carnitine treated diabetic rats. *Am. J. Physiol.* **245**: H969-H976, 1983.

24. Svabi F and Kirsch A. Diabetic type of cardiomyopathy in food restricted rats. *Can. J. Physiol. Pharm.* **70**: 1040-47, 1991.

25. Giacomelli F, Skazo L and Weiner J. Lysosomal enzymes in experimental diabetic cardiomyopathy. *Clin. Biochem.* **13**: 227-231, 1980.

26. Forgue ME and Freychet P. Insulin Receptors in the Heart Muscle: Demonstration of specific binding sites and impairment of insulin binding in the plasma membrane of the obese hyperglycemic mouse. *Diabetes* **24**: 715-723, 1975.

27. Malhotra A, Mjordes JP, McDermott L and Schaible T. Abnormal cardiac biochemistry in the spontaneouslydiabetic rat BB/W rat. *Am. J. Physiol.* **249**: H1051-H1055, 1985.

28. Garber DW, Evereet AW and Neely JR. Cardiac function and myosin ATPase in diabetic rats treated with insulin, T3 & T4. *Am. J. Physiol.* **244**: H592-H598, 1983.

29. Pittman CS, Suda AK, Chambers JB and Ray GY. Impaired 3,5,3,-triiodothyronine (t3) production in diabetic patients: *Metabolism* **28**: 333-338, 1979.

30. Galderisi M, Anderson KM, Wilson PWF and Levy D. Echocardiographic evidence of a distinct diabetic cardiomyopathy: the Framingham heart study. *Am. J. Cardiol.* **68**: 85-89, 1991.

31. William B, Levy K and Levy D. Diabetes, Glucose intolerance and left ventricular hypertrophy in the Framingham study. *J. Am. Coll. Cardiol.* **21**: 53A, 1993.

32. Mustonen J, Uusitupa MJ, Tahvanainen L, Talwar S, Laakso M, Lansimies E, Kuikka J and Pyorala K. Impaired Left ventricular systolic function during exercise in middle aged insulin dependent and non insulin dependent diabetic subjects without clinically evident cardiovascular disease. *Am J Cardiol.* **62**: 1273-1279.1988.

33. Avendano F, Jain A, Dharamsey S, Patel N, Reddi A and Regan TJ. The influence of moderate obesity on left ventricular diastolic functin in hypertension: Role of glucose and insulin. *Clin. Res.* **42**: 323A, 1994.

34. Vary TC and Neely JR. A mechanism for reduced myocardial Carnitine levels in diabetic animals. *Am. J. Physiol.* **243**: H154-H158, 1982.

35. Reibel DK, Wyse BW, Berkech DA and Neely JR. Regulation of coenzyme A synthesis in heart muscle: Effects of diabetes and fasting. *Am. J. Physiol.* **240**: H606-H611, 1981

36. Conlee RK and Tipton CM. Cardiac glycogen repletion after exercise. Influence of synthase and glucose 6 phosphate. *J. Appl. Physiol.* **42**: 240-244, 1974.

37. Neely JR and Morgan HE. Relationship between carbohydrate and lipid metabolism and the energy balance of heart muscles. *Ann. Rev. Physiol.* **36**: 413-459, 1974.

38. Ingebretsen WR, Peralta C, Monsher M, Wagner LK, and Ingebretsen C. Diabetes alters the myocardial cAMP-Protein Kinase Cascade System. *Am. J. Physiol.* **240**: H375-382, 1981.

39. Vadlamudi RVSV and McNeill JH. Effect of experimental diabctcs on ratc cardiac cAMP, Phosphorylasc, and inotropy. *Am J Physiol.* **244**: H844-H851, 1983.

40. Rannels DE, Jeffferson LS, Hjalmarson AC, Wolpert EB and Morgan HE. Maintenance of protein synthesis in hearts of diabetic animals. *Biochem Biophys Res Commun.* **40**: 1110-1116, 1970.

41. Whitman V, Schuler HG and Neely JR. Effect of alloxan induced diabetes on the hypertrophic response of rat heart. *J. Mol. Cell. Cardiol.* **11**: 1275-1281, 1979.

42. Senges J, Brachmann J, Pelzer D, Hasslacher C, Weihe E and Kubler W. Altered cardiac automaticity and conduction in experimental diabetes mellitus. *J. Mol. Cell. Cardiol.* **12**: 1341-1351, 1980.

43. Fein FS, Aronson RS, Nordin C, Miller-Green B and Sonnenblick EH. Altered myocardial response to ouabain in diabetic rats: mechanics and electrophysiology. *J. Mol. Cell. Cardiol.* **15**: 769-784, 1983

44. Shimoni Y, Firek L, Severson D and Giles W. Short term diabetes alters K^+ currents in rat ventricular myocytes. *Circ Res.* **74**: 620-628 ,1994.

45. Nordin C, Gilat E and Aronson RS: Delayed after depolarizations and triggered activity in ventricular muscle from ratswith streptozocin-induced diabetes. *Circ. Res.* **57**: 28-34, 1985.

46. Kneil PC, Junker U, Perrin IV, Bestetti GE and Rosi GHL. Varied effects of experimental diabetes on the autonomic nervous system of the rat. *Lab. Invest.* **54**: 523-530, 1986.

47. Uccioli L, Magnani P, Tilli P, Cotroneo P, Manto A, Greco AV, Sima AAF, Greene DA, Menzinger G and Ghirlanda G. Abnormal agonist stimulated cardiac parasympathetic acetylcholine release in streptozocin-induced diabetes. *Diabetes* **42**: 141-147, 1993.

48. Schimdt RE, Pleurad SB, Olack BJ and Scharp DW. The effect of pancreatic islet transplantationand insulin therapy on experimental diabetic autonomic neuropathy. *Diabetes* **32**: 532-540, 1983.

49. Yoshida T, Nishioka H, Yoshioka K, Nakano K, Dondo M and Terashima H. Effect of aldose reductase inhibitor ONO 2235 on reduced sympathetic nervous system activity and peripheral nerve disorders STZ-induced diabetic rats. *Diabetes* **36**: 6-13, 1987.

50. Knatterud GL, Klimt CR, Levin ME, Jacobson ME and Goldner MG. Effects of hypoglycemic agents on vascular complications in patients with adult onset diabetes: University group diabetes program VII. Mortality and selected nonfatal events with insulin treatment. *JAMA.* **240**: 37-42, 1978.

51. Kannel WB, Cupples LA, D'agostino RB and Stokes J: Hypertension, antihypertensive treatment and sudden coronary death: the Framingham study. *Hypertension* **11**:II-45-II-50.1988.

52. Bernardi L, Ricordi L, Lazzari P, Solda P, Calciati A, Ferrare MR, Vandea I, Finardi G, Fratino P. Impaired circadian modulation of sympathovagal activity in diabetes. A possible explanation for altered temporal onset of cardiovascular disease. *Circulation* **89**: 1443-1452, 1992.

53. Sampson MJ, Wilson S, Karagiannis P, Edmonds M, Watkins PJ. Progression of diabetic autonomic neuropathy over a

decade in insulin-dependent diabetics. *Quart. J. Med.* **278**: 635-646, 1990

54. Pierce GN and Dhalla NS. Sarcolemma Na$^+$-K$^+$ ATPase activity in diabetic rat heart. *Am. J. Physiol.* **245**: C241-247, 1983.

55. De Pover A, Grupp G, Schwartz A and Grupp I. Coupling of contraction through effect on Na,K-ATPase: Changes in Na,K-ATPase isoforms in heart disease. *Heart Failure* **6**: 201-211, 1991

56. Kjeldsen K. Braendgaard H, Sidenius P, Stenfatt LJ and Norgadd A. Diabetes decreses Na-K pump concentration in skeletal muscles, heart ventricular muscle, and peripheral nerves of rat. *Diabetes.* **36**: 842-848, 1987.

57. Tehrani ST, Yamamoto JJ and Garner MH. Na, K-ATPase and changes in ATP hydrolysis, monovalent cation afffinity and potassium occlusion in diabetic and galactosemic rats. *Diabetes* **39**: 1472-1478, 1990.

58. Moore RD. Effects of insulin upon ion transport. *Biochim. Biophys. Acta.* **737**: 1-49, 1983.

59. Lagadic-Grossman D, Chesnais JM and Feuvray D. Intracellular pN regulation in papillary muscles cells from streptozocin diabetic rats: An ion-sensitive microelectrode study. *Pfugers Arch.* **412**: 613-617, 1988.

60. Horakova M and Murphy MG. Effects of chronic diabetes mellitus on the electrical and contractile acivities, calcium transport,fatty acid profiles and ultrastructure of isolated rat ventricular myocytes. *Pflugers Arch.* **411**: 564-572, 1988.

61. Tani M and Neely JR. Hearts from diabetic rats are more resistant to in vitro ischemia: Possible role of altered Ca^{2+} metabolism. *Circ. Res.* **62**: 931-940, 1988

62. Bergh CH, Hjalmarson A, Sjogren KG and Jacobsson B. The effect of diabetes on phosphatidylinositol turnover and calcium influx in myocardium. *Horm. Metabol. Res.* **20**: 381-386, 1989.

63. Simmons DA and Winegrad AL. Mechanism of glucose induced Na-K ATPase inhibition in aortic wall of rabbits. *Diabetologia* **32**: 402-408, 1989.

64. Pugilise G, Tilton RG, Speedy A, Santarelli E, Eades DM, Province MA, Kilo C, Sherman WR and Williamson JR. Modulation of hemodynamic and vascular filtration changes in diabetic rats by dietary myoinositol. *Diabetes* **39**: 312-322, 1990.

65. Williamson JR, Chang K, Tilton RG, Prater C, Jeffrey JR, Weigel C, Sherman WR, Eades DM and Kilo C. Increased vascular permeability in spontaneously diabetic BB/W rats and in rats with mild versus severe streptozotocin induced diabetes. Prevention by aldose reductase inhibitors and castration. *Diabetes* **36**: 813-821, 1987.

66. Regan TJ, Beyer-Mears A, Torres R and Fusilli LD. Myocardial inositol and sodium in diabetes. *Int. Cardiol.* **37**: 309-316, 1992.

67. Schmidt RE, Plurad SB, Coleman BD, Williamson FR, and Tilton RG. Effects of sorbinil, dietary myo-inositol supplementation, and insulin on resolution of neuroaxonal dystrophy in mesenteric nerves of streptozocin-induced diabetic rats. *Diabetes.* **40**: 574-582, 1991.

68. Masuda Y and Levy MN. Heart rate modulates the disposition of neurallly released norepinephrine in cardiac tissues. *Circ. Res.* **57**: 19-27, 1985.

69. Lucas PD and Qirbi A. Tissue noradrenaline and the polyol pathway in experimentally diabetic rats. *Br. J. Pharmacol.* **97**: 347-352, 1989.

70. Gangully PK, Dhalla KS, Innes IR, Beamish RE and Dhalla NS. Altered norepinephrine turnover and metabolism in diabetic cardiomyopathy. *Circ. Res.* **59**: 684-693, 1986.

71. Ikstrup KM, Keane WF and Michels LD. Intravascular and extracellular volumes in the diabetic rat. *Life Sci.* **29**: 717-724, 1981.

72. Eisenhofer G, Smolich JJ, Cox NS and Esler MD. Neuronal reuptake of norepineprine and production of dihydroxyphenyglycol by cardiac sympathetic nerves in the anesthetized dog. *Circulation* **84**: 1354-1363, 1991.

73. Monckton G and Marusyk H. The effects of myoinositiol on the autonomic neuropathy in the streptozocin diabetic rat freeze-fracture study. *Can. J. Neurol. Sci.* **15**: 147-151, 1988.

74. Haider B, Lyons M, Torres R, Oldewortel H and Regan TJ. Effects of diabetes on myocardial perfusion in the athcrosclcrotic monkey. *J. Lab. Clin. Med.* **113**: 123-132, 1989.

75. Cohen RA. Dysfuncion of vascular endothelium in diabetes mellitus. *Circulation.* **87**: V67-V76, 1993.

76. Tilton RG, Chang K, Hasan KS, Smith SR, Petrash MJ, Misko TP, Moore WM, Currie MG, Corbett JA, McDaniel ML and Williamson JR. Prevention of diabetic vascular dysfunction by guanidines. *Diabetes* **42**: 221-232, 1993.

77. Nitenberg A, Valensi P, Saach R, Dali M, Aptecar E and Attali JR. Impairment of coronary vascular reserve and Ach-induced coronary vasodilation in diabetic patients with angiographically normal coronary arteries and normal left ventricular function. *Diabetes* **42**: 1017-1025, 1993.

78. Haider B, Ahmed SS, Moschos CB, Oldewurtel HA, Regan TJ. Myocardial function and coronary blood flow response to acute ischemia in chronic canine diabetes. *Circ. Res* **40**:577-583, 1977.

79. Singer DE, Moulton AW and Nathan DM: Diabetic myocardial infarction: interaction of diabetes with other preinfarction risk factors. *Diabetes* **38**: 350-357, 1989.

80. Mueller HS, Cohen LS, Braunwask E, Forman S, Feit F, Ross A, Schweiger M, Cabin H, Davison R, Miller D, Solomon R, Knatterud GL for the TIMI Investigators. Predictors of early morbidity and mortality after thrombolytic therapy of acute myocardial infarction. *Circulation* **85**: 1254-1264, 1992.

81. Sunni S, Bishop SP, Kent SP and Geer JC. Diabetic cardiomyopathy. *Arch. Pathol. Lab. Med.* **110**: 375-381, 1986.

CHAPTER 4

Therapeutic Interventions in the Diabetic Heart

John H. McNeill
Brian Rodrigues

Heart disease in chronic diabetes

Chronic diabetics in general have a higher incidence of and mortality from cardiac disease [1,2]. A wide spectrum of cardiac problems plague the chronic diabetic and include left-ventricular dilatation and hypertrophy, lower stroke volume and cardiac output and abnormalities of left-ventricular ejection time and prolongation of the pre-ejection period [3-5]. Although studies have shown that the incidence of causative factors such as large and small vessel disease and autonomic neuropathy [6] are increased during diabetes, these factors cannot always be definitely implicated as contributing agents to myocardial problems, due to their absence in a significant number of diabetic patients [7]. These results suggest that a specific cardiomyopathy may be a causal factor in producing the increase in mortality and morbidity of diabetes [8,9].

Although clinical studies give us some indication of the factors that may cause heart disease in diabetics, a better understanding can only be obtained from well-controlled experimental studies. The most commonly used models include alloxan or streptozotocin (STZ) induction of diabetes in dogs and rats. These drugs selectively destroy pancreatic ß-cells and produce a diabetic state, the severity of which can be varied by altering the dose of the agent. With time (about 4-6 weeks in the rat), animals so treated develop biochemical and functional myocardial abnormalities which appear to be a result of the drug induced hypoinsulinemia rather than a direct effect of the drug itself. Diminished ventricular compliance leading to underfilling and depressed contractility, stroke work and cardiac output have been reported in cardiac muscle preparations from these diabetic animals [10-14]. One problem with the above models is that they do not entirely resemble Type 1 insulin dependent diabetes mellitus (IDDM) [15]. Spontaneously diabetic (BB) rats are the closest counterpart to human IDDM [16]. If BB diabetic rats are maintained on a low dose of insulin, they also exhibit depressed left ventricular developed pressure, cardiac contractility and ventricular relaxation rates [17]. The above studies suggest that parallel to human findings, chronic diabetes mellitus in animals can negatively alter myocardial function independent of vascular defects.

Etiology of diabetic cardiomyopathy

Several etiological factors have been put forward to explain the development of diabetic cardiomyopathy and these include metabolic, ultrastructural and biochemical changes [for review see reference [18]; many of these issues are also covered in more detail in the other chapters in this book].

Metabolic alterations
In the early stages of diabetes, alterations in both fuel supply and utilization by the heart tissue may be the initiating factor for the development of diabetic cardiomyopathy [19].

Altered lipid metabolism -- Numerous human and animal studies have attempted to correlate changes in lipid and lipoprotein metabolism seen during diabetes to the observed excess in cardiovascular risk. In the heart, the source of cellular energy in the form of ATP is obtained via the oxidation of various substrates including free fatty acids (FFA), glucose, lactate and ketone bodies, with FFA being the principal substrate utilized by the heart. FFA are supplied to the heart from several sources: either through lipolysis of endogenous triglyceride stores or from the blood where they are carried as free acid bound to albumin or as triglyceride in chylomicrons and very low density lipoproteins. During diabetes, there is a marked increase in adipose tissue lipolysis with a subsequent outflow of FFA, which become greatly elevated in diabetic plasma [20]. When the rate of FFA uptake exceeds the rate of disposal, myocardial FFA levels and hence triglyceride content is increased [21]. FFA at high concentrations have been associated with a reduced cardiac contractile force and a greater susceptibility to arrhythmias in both control and diabetic hearts [22]. On the other hand, increased myocardial oxidation of FFA of endogenous or exogenous origin may have potentially deleterious consequences: an abnormally high requirement of oxygen for catabolism and an intracellular accumulation of potentially toxic intermediates of FFA metabolism. The involvement of these intermediates in diabetic heart failure is controversial. However, reports have suggested that these intermediates, if levels are sufficiently high, may have adverse electrophysiological, biochemical and mechanical effects on the heart. (The effect of diabetes on metabolism of FFA is discussed in Chapter 10.)

Altered carbohydrate metabolism -- Intracellular glucose disposal occurs through several major pathways. Nonoxidative glucose disposal primarily reflects the conversion to glycogen whereas the oxidative pathway involves either the complete oxidation of glucose-derived carbon atoms to carbon dioxide or the conversion to fatty acids in lipogenic tissues. Insulin affects all areas of carbohydrate metabolism, chiefly by controlling the transport of glucose. In insulin-responsive tissues, insulin controls the transport of glucose by facilitating the reversible translocation of glucose transporter proteins (GLUT 4) from a latent intracellular pool to the plasma membrane and a possible enhancement in the intrinsic activity of the transporters. Hence, in the hypoinsulinemic condition, there is a significant reduction in myocardial glucose utilization which probably results from a cellular depletion of GLUT 4 protein/activity [23]. Impaired glucose metabolism can also result from excessive myocardial FFA oxidation [21,24-27]. (The alterations in glycogen and glucose metabolism are discussed in Chapters 8 and 9 respectively)

Ultrastructural changes

Hearts from chronically diabetic rats were observed to have mitochondrial clumping and disruption with intramitochondrial dense staining particles, loss of contractile protein and disrupted banding, sarcolemmal and sarcoplasmic reticular changes, edematous focal areas adjacent to the sarcoplasmic reticulum, capillary changes like thickening of lamina densa, loss of lamina lucida and an increased number of micropinocytic vesicles in the capillary walls and increased lipid levels [19]. The above changes were paralleled by a depression in cardiac function. With a progressive deterioration in myocardial ultrastructure, there was no further worsening of cardiac performance [28]. McGrath *et al.* [29] subsequently demonstrated that some, but not all, of the above ultrastructural changes could be reversed by insulin treatment.

Biochemical changes

Various biochemical changes in the myocardium have also been characterized in animal models of diabetes. The more prominent systems affected, which are known to regulate calcium homeostasis and hence cardiac function, are the sarcolemma and sarcoplasmic reticulum [30]. Several studies in experimental diabetes have demonstrated myocardial sarcolemmal defects such as an increased permeability, thickening of glycocalyx (due to alterations in sialic acid synthesis in the basement membrane), depressed Na^+-K^+-ATPase and adenylate cyclase activities and defective Na^+-Ca^{2+}-exchanger and Ca^{2+}-pump [30].

The sarcoplasmic reticulum (SR) acts as a calcium store which is capable of releasing and taking up calcium on a beat-to-beat basis, thus promoting contraction and relaxation of myofibrils [31]. Our laboratory has demonstrated that in diabetic rats, depressed cardiac SR calcium uptake may be due to the inhibition of Ca^{2+}-ATPase [32]. In a recent report from our laboratory, Yu *et al.* [33] using isolated diabetic cardiac myocytes demonstrated that SR calcium content was decreased.

Another prominent system closely associated with contractility, which is altered by diabetes, are the contractile proteins. A number of studies have shown that the isoenzyme distribution shifts from the normally predominant V_1 form to the less active V_3 form in diabetic rats with a corresponding decrease in Ca^{2+}-ATPase activities of myosin and actomyosin. This could

69

then account for the decreased shortening velocity of cardiac muscle. Mitochondrial changes like decreased oxidative capacity and Mg^{2+}-ATPase and calcium uptake activity have also been implicated as playing a crucial role in the development of diabetic cardiomyopathy [30]. (Chapters 3, 5 and 6 address these and other biochemical alterations due to diabetes.)

Therapeutic interventions in the diabetic heart

Research in our laboratory initially made attempts to develop measures to prevent or reverse the entire diabetic state. Subsequently, measures targeting more selective changes were developed. The treatment protocols used were as follows:

Insulin and insulin-mimicking agents

Insulin -- The most successful therapeutic intervention in preventing and reversing the secondary complications associated with diabetes is insulin treatment. If STZ diabetic rats were treated with insulin for 6 weeks (10 U kg^{-1} protamine zinc insulin, s.c. daily) immediately after they were injected with STZ, there was a normalization of cardiac function. If cardiac function was first allowed to decrease in animals by allowing them to remain diabetic, the heart function could also be reversed to normal by 4 weeks of insulin treatment. However, if rats were made diabetic for 6 months and then treated for 4 weeks with insulin, cardiac function was only partially restored suggesting that either the changes at these chronic stages of diabetes are irreversible or that the insulin treatment protocol was inadequate for complete normalization [34].

Vanadium -- Although insulin treatment prevents and reverses diabetes-induced myocardial alterations in rats, major problems with insulin treatment clinically include hypoglycemia, inadequate control in some diabetics and the persistence of secondary complications. It would thus be desirable and useful to have drug treatments which could either substitute for insulin or could be used in addition to the peptide in preventing diabetes-induced myocardial alterations. It had been reported that vanadium exhibits several *in vitro* insulin-mimetic properties [35,36]. When vanadate was administered for a 4-week period to diabetic rats in their drinking water, their blood glucose was not significantly different from that of nondiabetic controls despite a low plasma insulin. In addition, cardiac performance was depressed in the untreated diabetic animals, but the cardiac performance of the vanadate-treated diabetic animals was not significantly different from that of nondiabetic controls [37,38]. Interestingly, the improvements in plasma glucose and cardiac performance in these animals were not associated with an increase in plasma insulin. In fact, vanadate was found to decrease plasma insulin in control animals, an observation which has been attributed to its insulin-enhancing properties. Similar effects of vanadium in improving the diabetic state have been reported in partially pancreatectomized and spontaneously diabetic BB/W rats and genetically obese and hyperinsulinemic *fa/fa* rats and *ob/ob* mice.

Oral vanadium in the form of vanadyl (+4 oxide form) has also been demonstrated to be effective in lowering glucose and improving heart function in STZ-diabetic rats [39]. Using vanadyl, an interesting feature observed was that plasma glucose and cardiac performance remained improved in treated diabetic rats after vanadyl treatment had been withdrawn for 13 weeks [40]. Subsequently, it was demonstrated that in these vanadyl treated diabetic rats from which treatment had been withdrawn for several weeks, there was an improved islet insulin content and normal fasting plasma insulin levels [41]. We have also administered oral vanadyl sulfate to spontaneously diabetic BB/W rats [42] and observed that although treatment did not completely remove the animals dependence on insulin, it significantly reduced insulin requirement to maintain euglycemia.

As oral vanadate and vanadyl have local side effects like diarrhea and limited absorption from the gastrointestinal tract [43], our laboratory has been developing more orally potent forms of vanadyl in an attempt to lower the incidence of gastrointestinal toxicity. Two organic vanadyl derivatives tested and found to have potent antidiabetic properties were naglivan (Bis(cysteine,amide N-octyl)oxovanadium IV) and BMOV (Bis(maltolato)oxovanadium IV) [44-48]. Treatment of diabetic rats with either of these compounds prevented the diabetes induced decrease in heart function.

Sodium selenate -- Selenium has been demonstrated to possess insulin-like actions. Rat adipocytes incubated with sodium selenate demonstrated a markedly increased glucose transport [49]. In our laboratory, STZ-diabetic rats treated with sodium selenate for 7 weeks showed a decrease in plasma glucose to control levels. Plasma insulin was reduced in control rats given sodium selenate to the level found in the diabetic and treated diabetic rats. Thus, the actions of sodium selenate, when administered *in vivo*, are similar to those of vanadium and insulin [50].

Interventions which affect lipid metabolism

Carnitine -- In order for fatty acids to be oxidized, they must be transported across the inner mitochondrial membrane. Carnitine acts as a cofactor, allowing acyl groups to be shuttled between intramitochondrial and extramitochondrial pools of CoA and hence adequate levels are required for energy production. Carnitine is also capable of storing, transporting and excreting potentially toxic acyl compounds, by facilitating their conversion to acylcarnitines, when the metabolic system malfunctions or is overloaded. Unlike the corresponding acyl CoA, acyl carnitines can diffuse out of the cell into the blood stream. Urinary clearances for the potentially toxic acylcarnitines are 10- to 20-fold higher than for free carnitine; therefore excess amounts of serum acylcarnitine can be rapidly eliminated by the kidneys.

When the carnitine level in tissues is increased, the pre-existing acetyl-CoA is transformed into acetyl carnitine which can then either a) remain as a storage depot, b) be converted into fatty acid or cholesterol or c) cross the mitochondrial membrane back to the cytosol and from there into the circulation to be eventually excreted in the urine. An important consequence of this effect of carnitine is that it serves as a buffer of the metabolically critical acetyl CoA pool and hence decreases the intramitochondrial acetyl CoA/CoA ratio. A decrease in this ratio increases pyruvate dehydrogenase activity leading to an increase in glucose oxidation.

As carnitine plays such an important role in myocardial substrate utilization in the control heart, a cardiac sensitivity to depletion of carnitine (as seen during diabetes) is understandable. Lack of sufficient carnitine may be a factor responsible for inadequate entry of long-chain fatty acids into the mitochondrial matrix and hence an impaired utilization. This leads to an accumulation within the plasma or cytosol of FFA and/or a number of intermediates involved in FFA oxidation (e.g. acyl CoA) which, if sufficiently large, may disrupt myocardial cell function

It is evident, therefore, that adequate levels of carnitine are required for normal FFA and energy metabolism in heart muscle, and that changes in the levels of carnitine may affect energy production and muscle performance. We have administered carnitine to rats from the onset of diabetes to see whether this intervention could replenish total myocardial carnitine levels and possibly prevent the depression in heart after chronic diabetes. L-carnitine treatment of diabetic rats significantly increased myocardial carnitine levels, reduced plasma glucose and triglycerides and significantly improved diabetic cardiac performance [51].

Choline and Methionine -- During diabetes, there is an abnormal build-up of lipids in the myocardium. Choline and methionine have been used to control myocardial lipid accumulation as they are lipotropic agents and have been reported to modify the incidence of myocardial lesions in rats fed various fat diets. STZ diabetic rats were fed choline (0.3 mg/ml) and methionine (0.25 mg/ml) in their drinking water for 7 weeks. Myocardial levels of cholesterol and triglycerides when measured, were found to be reduced in the treated diabetic animals. In addition, cardiac performance was depressed in untreated diabetic animals, but there was a significant improvement in heart function in treated diabetics relative to the untreated ones. Thus, it appeared that if the build-up of cholesterol and triglycerides in the diabetic myocardium could be controlled, the cardiac dysfunction which frequently accompanies this disease state can be modified. The mechanisms of choline and methionine in reducing the elevated myocardial cholesterol and triglycerides in the diabetic heart are a matter of speculation. These two lipotropic agents are involved in the synthesis of phosphatidylcholine which provides an integral part of the structure and assembly system of lipoproteins and bile salt micelles which play a strategic role in cholesterol transport. Furthermore, choline is involved in carnitine synthesis, and as previously stated, reduced myocardial carnitine levels are observed during diabetes [52].

Hydralazine -- Hydralazine, a vasodilator used for the treatment of hypertension and congestive heart failure has one unusual property and that is its ability to lower blood lipids. We therefore investigated whether hydralazine could lower plasma triglycerides and alleviate the mechanical dysfunction associated with chronic diabetes. In STZ-diabetic rats, hydralazine had triglyceride-lowering properties and was capable of preventing the cardiodepressant effect of diabetes. The improvement in cardiac function by hydralazine could not be explained on the basis of its direct actions on the heart [53].

It is unclear as to why triglyceride levels are decreased in the hydralazine-treated diabetic rats, even when they lack insulin. It is possible that hydralazine, like insulin, inhibits adipose tissue lipolysis. To determine if the mechanism of action of hydralazine as a lipid lowering agent occurred at the site of adipose tissue, the *in vitro* effects of hydralazine were tested in adipose tissue from control and diabetic rats. The results indicated that hydralazine had no effect on the basal release of glycerol from adipose tissue which remained elevated in the diabetic rats [54]. Another possible explanation for the decrease in plasma lipids is that the metabolic changes observed in untreated diabetes are, in many respects, similar to those produced by the infusion of catecholamines. Indeed, isoproterenol, used as the lipolytic stimulus, increases glycerol output from both control and diabetic adipose tissue. Thus, the absence of elevated plasma lipids in the hydralazine-treated diabetic rats could be due to a direct effect of hydralazine on the action of catecholamines. However, we have reported that hydralazine does not reduce the isoproterenol induced glycerol release at any concentration, in control and diabetic rats [54]. It could hence be concluded that the triglyceride lowering effect of hydralazine does not occur at the site of the adipose tissue. Whether hydralazine may directly influence the rate of lipid or lipoprotein biosynthesis in the liver is as yet unknown. However, the liver is the major site of metabolism of hydralazine and it is possible that a relationship exists between the metabolism of hydralazine and hepatic lipid synthesis.

Thyroid hormone -- Fifty percent of overtly hypothyroid patients demonstrate decreased clearance of both endogenous and exogenous triglycerides [55]. This may be secondary to decreased lipoprotein lipase activity. Lipid analyses also reveal diminished turnover of LDL cholesterol and significantly elevated LDL-to-HDL cholesterol ratios [56]. Diabetes is known to have a number of cardiac mechanical and biochemical effects similar to those seen in hypothyroidism, such as depressed force-velocity relaxation in papillary muscles, depressed calcium transport by the sarcoplasmic reticulum and actomyosin Ca^{2+}-ATPase activities, a shift in the myosin isozyme subtype distributions from the "fast" V_1 form to the "slow" V_3 form as well as altered lipid metabolism. Diabetes has also been known to induce hypothyroidism (reduced levels of plasma T_3 or thyroxine). It is thus possible that diabetes-induced myocardial alterations could be a result of the hypothyroidism which is seen in diabetes [17]. Consequently, we investigated whether the diabetes-induced functional and biochemical changes are preventable by thyroid replacement therapy. However, thyroid hormone treatment did not prove to be an effective method for normalizing lipid changes or myocardial function in diabetic rats [57]. Using pharmacological doses of thyroid hormones to treat diabetic rats, Dillman [58] had previously reported that the isoenzyme shift in diabetic hearts was at least partially reversible. Hence, we treated diabetic rats with a combination of thyroid hormone and myoinositol (a lipotropic agent) and found that such a treatment improved diabetic heart function and this coincided with a significant decrease in the myocardial triacylglycerol levels [59]. Similarly, a combination of thyroid hormone and methyl palmoxirate (which inhibits fatty acid oxidation, lowers blood glucose levels in diabetic rats and prevents the depression in SR calcium uptake) was able to improve diabetic heart function [60].

Plasma triglycerides and diabetic heart function --The above studies attempted to correlate myocardial alterations in diabetic rats to alterations in lipid metabolism. We therefore decided to investigate the relationship between plasma lipids and heart function in the diabetic rat, using other agents which are known to reduce plasma triglyceride levels. Hence, the beneficial effects of clofibrate, verapamil and prazosin administration were studied in diabetic rats. Although these treatments lowered plasma triglycerides, at least at the doses used, they did not prevent diabetic cardiomyopathy from occurring. It should be pointed out

75

that our results obtained with verapamil are in contrast to those reported by Afzal *et al*. [61,62]. These authors concluded that verapamil treatment was capable of partially preventing the diabetes-induced changes in heart function, metabolism, enzyme activity and ultrastructure. The discrepancy observed between the two studies with respect to the ability of verapamil to improve cardiac function could reflect differences in methodology. In the experiments of Afzal *et al*. [61,62] cardiac function was measured in *in vivo* anesthetized rats, whereas our studies were done on isolated perfused rat hearts *in vitro*. In summary, our studies suggest that in the chronically diabetic rat, hypertriglyceridemia alone may not be as important as previously suggested in the development of cardiac dysfunction. It appears more likely that improving myocardial glucose utilization is more critical than triglyceride lowering, in preventing cardiac dysfunction in the diabetic rat [54].

Interventions which affect carbohydrate metabolism

Alterations in glucose oxidation in the diabetic heart could be a significant causative factor in the development of diabetic cardiomyopathy. Impaired glucose oxidation could result from a depletion of glucose transporters or a decreased rate of glucose phosphorylation. The latter in turn could result from the increased metabolism of FFA. Thus agents which inhibit oxidation of fatty acids (e.g. 2-tetradecylglycidic acid; 2[5(4-chlorophenyl) pentyl oxirane-2-carboxylic acid; etomoxir; B 827-33) have been shown to be effective hypoglycemic agents in STZ-diabetic animals [for review see ref. 20]. We studied the effect of agents which affect glucose utilization (either directly or via an effect on fatty acid utilization) on cardiac dysfunction in diabetic rats.

Dichloroacetate -- Dichloroacetate (DCA) is a pyruvate dehydrogenase complex activator that is effective in increasing myocardial glucose oxidation in normal and diabetic rat hearts. Therefore, we examined cardiac performance in FFA perfused hearts from short (6 weeks) and long (24 weeks) term diabetic rats through which DCA was recirculated. Addition of DCA to palmitate-perfused, spontaneously beating hearts from short term diabetic rats resulted in an acute improvement in cardiac function. Addition of DCA to hearts from long term diabetic rats resulted in

76

only a small improvement in heart function and probably reflects the onset of irreversible changes in cardiac function at this time point [63].

Metformin -- This agent lowers fasting glucose levels and improves glucose tolerance in diabetic patients without eliciting an increase in insulin levels. We studied the effects of metformin in preventing diabetic cardiomyopathy in STZ diabetic rats. Treatment with metformin lowered plasma glucose levels in diabetic rats and improved cardiac function [64].

Conclusion

The occurrence of cardiovascular diseases is much greater in diabetic patients. The factors responsible are multifactorial. We propose that the cardiac defects could result because of the following sequence of events. Abnormalities in myocardial metabolism first occur as a result of hypoinsulinemia and may provide the initial biochemical lesion from which further events ensue. These include the accumulation of metabolic intermediates which could cause abnormalities in calcium homeostasis either directly, or indirectly through structural and functional subcellular membrane alterations. The latter include depressed myosin ATPase, Na^+-K^+ ATPase and Ca^{2+}-ATPase activity as well as decreased sarcoplasmic reticulum calcium transport. From the point of view of therapeutic intervention, therapies which target cardiac metabolic aberrations during the initial stages of diabetes can potentially delay or impede the progression of more permanent sequelae and can prevent diabetic heart disease.

Acknowledgments

Some of the studies described in this paper were supported by grants from the B.C. and Yukon Heart Foundation, MRC (Canada), the B.C. Health Research Foundation and the Canadian Diabetes Association. BR is a Canadian Diabetes Association Research Scholar.

References

1. Kannel WB and McGee DL. Diabetes and cardiovascular disease: The Framingham Study. *JAMA* **241**: 2035-2038, 1979.

2. Palumbo PJ, Elveback CR and Conolly DC. Coronary artery disease and congestive heart failure in the diabetic: Epidemiological aspects. The Rochester Diabetes Project. In *Clinical Cardiology and Diabetes*, Scott RC, Ed., Futura, New York, p. 13, 1981.

3. Hamby RI, Zoneraich S and Sherman L. Diabetic cardiomyopathy. *JAMA* **229**: 1749-1754, 1974.

4. Regan TJ, Lyons MM and Ahmed SS. Evidence for cardiomyopathy in familial diabetes mellitus. *J. Clin. Invest.* **60**: 885-889, 1977.

5. D'Elia JA, Weinrauch LA, Healy RW, Libertino RW, Bradley RF and Leland OS. Myocardial dysfunction without coronary artery disease in diabetic renal failure. *Am. J. Cardiol.* **43**: 193-199, 1979.

6. Ledet B, Neubauer B, Christensen NJ, Lundback K. Diabetic cardiopathy. *Diabetologia* **16**: 207-209, 1979.

7. Ahmed SS, Jaferi GA, Narang RM and Regan TJ. Preclinical abnormality of left ventricular function in diabetes mellitus. *Am. Heart J.* **89**: 153-158, 1975.

8. Fein FS and Sonnenblick EH. Diabetic cardiomyopathy. *Prog. Cardiovasc. Res.* **27**: 255-270, 1985.

9. Galderisi M, Anderson KM, Wilson PWF and Levy D. Echocardiographic evidence for the existence of a distinct diabetic cardiomyopathy (The Framingham Heart Study). *Am. J. Cardiol.* **68**: 85-89, 1991.

10. Regan TJ, Ettinger PO, Khan MI, Jesran MU, Lyons MM, Oldewurtel HA and Weber M. Altered myocardial function and metabolism in chronic diabetes mellitus without ischemia in dogs. *Circ. Res.* **35**: 222-237, 1974.

11. Miller TB. Cardiac performance of isolated perfused hearts from alloxan diabetic rats. *Am. J. Physiol.* **236**: 808-812, 1979.

12. Vadllamudi RVSV, Rodgers RL and McNeill JH. The effect of chronic alloxan- and streptozotocin-induced diabetes on isolated rat heart performance. *Can. J. Physiol. Pharmacol.* **60**: 902-911, 1982.

13. Fein FS, Kornstein LB, Strobeck JE, Capasso JM and Sonnenblick EH. Altered myocardial mechanics in diabetic rats. *Circ. Res.* **47**: 922-933, 1980.

14. Rodrigues B and McNeill JH. Cardiac function in spontaneously hypertensive diabetic rats. *Am. J. Physiol.* **251**: 571-580, 1986.

15. National Diabetes Data Group. Classification and diagnosis of diabetes mellitus and other categories of glucose intolerance. *Diabetes* **28**: 1039-1057, 1979.

16. Marliss EB, Nakhooda AF, Poussier P and Sima AAF. The diabetic syndrome of the "BB" Wistar rat: Possible relevance to Type 1 (insulin-dependent) diabetes in man. *Diabetologia* **22**: 225-232, 1982.

17. Rodrigues B and McNeill JII. Cardiac dysfunction in isolated perfused hearts from spontaneously diabetic BB rats. *Can. J. Physiol. Pharmacol.* **68**: 514-518, 1990.

18. Rodrigues B and McNeill JH. The diabetic heart: metabolic causes for the development of a cardiomyopathy. *Cardiovas. Res.* **26**: 913-922, 1992.

19. Jackson CV, McGarth GM, Tahiliani AG, Vadlamudi RVSV and McNeill JH. A functional and ultrastructural analysis of experimental diabetic rat myocardium: Manifestation of cardiomyopathy. *Diabetes* **34**: 876-883, 1985.

20. Rodrigues B, Cam MC and McNeill JH. Myocardial substrate metabolism: Implications for diabetic cardiomyopathy. *J. Mol. Cell. Cardiol.* **27**: 169-179, 1995.

21. Chattopadhyay J, Thompson EW and Schmid HHO. Elevated levels of non-esterified fatty acids in the myocardium of alloxan diabetic rats. *Lipids* **25**: 307-310, 1990.

22. Opie L.H. Effect of fatty acid on contractility and rhythm of the heart. *Nature (Lond.)* **227**: 1055-1056, 1970.

23. Garvey WG, Hardin G, Juhaszova M and Dominguez JH. Effects of diabetes on myocardial glucose transport system in rats: Implication for diabetic cardiomyopathy. *Am. J. Physiol.* **264**: 837-844, 1993.

24. Randle PJ, Hales CN, Garland PB and Newsholme EA. The glucose fatty acid cycle: Its role in insulin sensitivity and the metabolic disturbances of diabetes mellitus. *Lancet* **1**: 785-789, 1963.

25. Kerby AK, Vary TC and Randle PJ. Molecular mechanisms regulating myocardial glucose oxidation. *Basic. Res. Cardiol.* **80** (Suppl 2): 93-96, 1985.

26. Wall SR and Lopaschuk GD. Glucose oxidation rates in fatty acid perfused isolated working hearts from diabetic rats. *Biochim. Biophys. Acta* **1006**: 97-103, 1989.

27. Chen V, Ianuzzo CD, Fong BC and Spitzer JJ. The effects of acute and chronic diabetes on myocardial metabolism in rats. *Diabetes* **33**:1078-1084, 1984.

28. Vadlamudi RVSV, Rodgers RL and McNeill JH. The effect of chronic alloxan- and streptozotocin-induced diabetes on isolated rat heart performance. *Can. J. Physiol. Pharmacol.* **60**: 902-911, 1982.

29. McGarth GM and McNeill JH. Cardiac ultrastructural changes in streptozotocin-induced diabetic rats: Effects of insulin treatment. *Can. J. Cardiol.* **2**:164-169, 1986.

30. Heyliger CE, Rodrigues B and McNeill JH. Alterations of cardiac muscle membranes in hypertension and diabetes mellitus. In *Membrane Abnormalities in Hypertension and Diabetes Mellitus*. Kwan CY (Ed), CRC Press Inc., Florida, pp.91-116, 1989.

31. Lopaschuk GD, Eibschutz B, Katz S and McNeill JH. Depression of calcium transport in sarcoplasmic reticulum from diabetic rats: Lack of involvement by specific regulatory mediators. *Gen. Pharmac.* **15**: 1-5, 1984.

32. Lopaschuk GD, Katz S and McNeill JH. The effect of alloxan- and streptozotocin-induced diabetes on calcium transport in rat cardiac sarcoplasmic reticulum. The possible involvement

of long chain acylcarnitines. *Can. J. Physiol. Pharmacol.* **61**: 439-448, 1983.

33. Yu Z, Tibbits GF and McNeill JH. Cellular function of diabetic cardiomyocytes: Contractility, rapid cooling contracture, and ryanodine binding. *Am. J. Physiol.* **266**: 2082-2089, 1994.

34. McNeill JH and Tahiliani AG. Diabetes-induced cardiac changes. *Trends Pharmacol. Sci.* **7**: 364-367, 1986.

35. Tolman EL, Barris E, Burns M, Prasini A and Partridge R. Effects of vanadium on glucose metabolism in vitro. *Life Sci.* **25**: 1159-1164, 1979.

36. Tamura S, Brown TA, Dubler RE and Larner. Insulin-like effect of vanadate on adipocyte glycogen synthase and on phosphorylation of 95,000 dalton subunit of insulin receptor. *Biochem. Biophys. Res. Commun.* **113**: 80-86, 1983.

37. Heyliger CE, Tahiliani AG and McNeill JH. Effect of vanadate on elevated blood glucose and depressed cardiac performance of diabetic rats. *Science* **227**: 1474-1477, 1985.

38. Takada K, Temma K and Akera T. Inotropic effects of vanadate in isolated rat and guinea-pig heart under conditions which modify calcium pools involved in contractile activation. *J. Pharmacol. Exp. Ther.* **222**: 132-139, 1982.

39. Ramanadham S, Mongold JJ, Brownsey RW, Cros GH and McNeill JH. Oral vanadyl sulfate in treatment of diabetes mellitus in rats. *Am. J. Physiol.* **257**: 904-911, 1989.

40. Ramanadham S, Brownsey RW, Cros GH, Mongold JJ and McNeill JH. Sustained prevention of myocardial and metabolic abnormalities in diabetic rats following withdrawal from oral vanadyl treatment. *Metabolism* **38**: 1022-1028, 1989.

41. Pederson RA, Ramanadham S, Buchan AMJ and McNeill JH. Long-term effects of vanadyl treatment on streptozocin-induced diabetes in rats. *Diabetes* **38**: 1390-1393, 1989.

42. Battell ML, Yuen VG and McNeill JH. Treatment of BB rats with vanadyl sulphate. *Pharmacol. Commun.* **1**: 291-301, 1992.

43. Underwood EJ. Vanadium. In Trace elements in human and animal nutrition. Academic Press, New York, pp 388-397, 1977.

44. Cam MC, Cros GH, Serrano JJ, Lazaro R and McNeill JH. In vivo antidiabetic actions of naglivan, an organic compound in streptozotocin-induced diabetes. *Diab. Res. Clin. Prac.* **20**: 11-121, 1993.

45. McNeill JH, Yuen VG, Hoveyda HR and Orvig C. Bis(maltolato)oxovanadium(IV) is a potent insulin mimic. *J. Med. Chem.* **35**: 1489-1491, 1992.

46. Ramanadham S, Cros GH, Mongold JJ, Serrano JJ, McNeill JH. Enhanced in vivo sensitivity of vanadyl-treated diabetic rats to insulin. *Can. J. Physiol. Pharmacol.* **68**: 486-491, 1990.

47. Yuen VG, Orvig C, Thompson KH and McNeill JH. Improvement in cardiac dysfunction in strepotozotocin-induced diabetic rats following chronic oral administration of bis(maltolato)oxovanadium(IV). *Can. J. Physiol. Pharmacol.* **71**: 270-276, 1992.

48. Yuen VG, Orvig C and McNeill JH. Comparison of the glucose lowering properties vanadyl sulfate and bis(maltolato)oxovanadium(IV) following acute and chronic administration. *Can. J. Physiol. Pharmacol.* (submitted).

49. Ezaki O. The insulin-like effects of selenate in rat adipocytes. *J. Biol. Chem.* **265**:1124-1128, 1990.

50. McNeill JH, Delgatty HLM and Battell ML. Insulin like effects of sodium selenate in streptozotocin-induced diabetic rats. *Diabetes* **40**: 1675-1678, 1991.

51. Rodrigues B, Xiang H and McNeill JH. Effect of L-carnitine treatment on lipid metabolism and cardiac performance in chronically diabetic rats. *Diabetes* **37**: 1358-1364, 1988.

52. Heyliger CE, Rodrigues B and McNeill JH. Effect of choline and methionine treatment on cardiac dysfunction of diabetic rats. *Diabetes* **35**: 1152-1157, 1986.

53. Rodrigues B, Goyal RK and McNeill JH. Effects of hydralazine on streptozotocin-induced diabetic rats:

prevention of hyperlipidemia and improvement in cardiac function. *J. Pharmacol. Exp. Ther.* **237**: 292-299, 1986.

54. Rodrigues B, Grassby PF, Battell ML, Lee SYN and McNeill JH. Hypertriglyceridemia in experimental diabetes: relationship to cardiac dysfunction. *Can. J. Physiol. Pharmacol.* **72**: 447-455, 1994.

55. Tulloch BR, Lewis B and Fraser TR. Triglyceride metabolism in thyroid disease. *Lancet* **1**: 391-394, 1973.

56. DeMartino GN and Goldberg AL. A possible explanation for myxedema and hypercholesterolemia in hypothyroidism. *Enzyme* **26**:1-7, 1981.

57. Tahiliani AG and McNeill JH. Lack of effect of thyroid hormone on diabetic rat heart function and biochemistry. *Can. J. Physiol. Pharmacol.* **62**: 617-621, 1984.

58. Dillman WH. Influence of thyroid hormone on myosin ATPase activity and myosin isoenzyme distribution in the heart of diabetic rats. *Metabolism* **31**:199-204, 1982.

59. Xiang H, Heyliger CE and McNeill JH. Effect of myo-Inositol and T_3 on myocardial lipids and cardiac function in streptozotocin-induced diabetic rats. *Diabetes* **37**: 1542-1548, 1988.

60. Tahiliani AG and McNeill JH. Prevention of diabetes-induced myocardial dysfunction in rats by methyl palmoxirate and triiodothyronine treatment. *Can. J. Physiol. Pharmacol.* **63**: 925-931, 1985.

61. Afzal N. Ganguly PK, Dhalla KS, Pierce GN, Singal PK and Dhalla NS. Beneficial effects of verapamil in diabetic cardiomyopathy. *Diabetes* **37**: 936-942, 1988.

62. Afzal N. Pierce GN, Elimban V, Beamish RE and Dhalla NS. Influence of verapamil on some subcellular defects in diabetic cardiomyopathy. *Am. J. Physiol.* **256**: 453-458, 1989.

63. Nicholl TA, Lopaschuk GD and McNeill JH. Effects of free fatty acids and dichloroacetate on isolated working diabetic rat heart. *Am. J. Physiol.* **261**: 1053-1059, 1991.

64. Verma S and McNeill JH. Metformin improves cardiac function in isolated streptozotocin-diabetic rat hearts. *Am. J. Physiol.* **266**: 714-719, 1994.

CHAPTER 5

Effect of Diabetes on Protein Synthesis in the Myocardium

David L. Geenen
Ashwani Malhotra

<u>**Measurements of protein synthesis, degradation and turnover in muscle**</u>

Protein turnover in muscle represents the net result of synthesis of new protein from a precursor pool of amino acids and the degradation of contractile, regulatory and other proteins into their constituent amino acids. In muscle, an array of hormonal, mechanical, and metabolic factors influence protein synthesis and degradation. Insulin, for example, is a potent stimulus of protein turnover increasing synthesis and attenuating degradation [1,2]. Fractional synthesis (K_s) and degradation (K_d) rate represent the fraction of the available precursor that is synthesized into protein or the protein product which is degraded into amino acids, respectively. Fractional synthesis rate is often expressed as a percent of the amino acid precursor pool utilized over time.

Several different methods are employed to assess protein synthesis *in vitro* and *in vivo* but a full description is beyond the scope of this chapter. The basic premise is that radiolabeled amino acids can be infused intravascularly or into a perfusion medium and subsequently equilibrate with the immediate precursor to protein, aminoacyl transfer RNA (tRNA). If the specific activities of the tracer amino acid in the precursor pool and the muscle protein are measured over the infusion period, the fractional synthesis rate and protein synthetic rate can be calculated. Since the aminoacyl tRNA is present in small quantities within muscle and acylated amino acids turnover rapidly, plasma specific activity of the tracer amino acid is used as an indicator of the precursor pool.

A number of studies report total cardiac protein synthesis data derived from radiolabeled amino acid infusion *in vivo*. Myosin heavy chain, actin, troponin, and tropomyosin all have different turnover rates [3-5], therefore, caution should be exercised when interpreting total cardiac protein synthesis data as reflecting protein synthesis of individual contractile proteins in the sarcomere.

The two most frequently used methods of measuring protein synthesis discussed in this chapter are the "flooding" and continuous infusion techniques [6]. The flooding technique is used most frequently under conditions in which the precursor amino acid pool is not expected to be in steady-state, such as during increased hormonal levels or hemodynamic load. Administration of the tracer in the flooding technique is easier than with continuous infusion since a single bolus infusion is required compared to multiple sampling. It is important to note that with the flooding technique, which requires a large amount of unlabeled amino acid infused along with the tracer, the specific radioactivity of the tracer is reduced and can complicate the protein synthetic analysis of individual cardiac contractile proteins such as myosin and actin. The continuous infusion technique allows for a more accurate determination of the precursor pool specific activity since infusion takes place over a longer period of time and allows for greater equilibration between the tracer and aminoacyl tRNA. Unlike protein synthesis, measurements of protein degradation cannot be derived as easily from amino acid tracer studies *in vivo* since amino acid reutilization complicates measurements of the radiolabeled tracer. Protein degradation can be estimated by taking the difference between protein synthesis and protein accumulation. This equation has inherent problems however, since protein synthesis is usually measured over a period of minutes to hours whereas protein accumulation in measurable quantities takes place over a period of days.

Protein turnover is also influenced by the RNA/protein ratio, defined as synthetic capacity, and the amount of protein synthesized per day relative to the amount of RNA (efficiency of protein synthesis). Following activation of intracellular precursor amino acids, protein is synthesized in a series of reactions which involve initiation and elongation of peptide chains. Peptide chain initiation is characterized by binding of messenger RNA (mRNA) and methionyl tRNA to the ribosomal subunits 40S and 60S. Elongation of the peptide chain represents further addition of activated amino acids dictated by mRNA. Both peptide chain initiation and elongation are modulated by specific intracellular factors which will be discussed below.

The effects of insulin on protein turnover

Studies of the heart *in vitro* demonstrate that insulin stimulates protein synthesis and inhibits protein degradation [7-9]. However less is known about the role of insulin in protein turnover in the intact myocardium. The effects of insulin or hyperinsulinemia on protein degradation has been studied in a number of different animal models [10-13]. In 36-hour fasted dogs, rates of myocardial protein synthesis and degradation, assessed *in vivo*, were unchanged during insulin and glucose infusion and were accompanied by a decline in amino acid concentrations [14]. When dogs received an infusion of amino acids along with normal glucose and insulin levels within the first 16 hours of fasting, protein degradation was inhibited by 50% suggesting that the effect of insulin on maintaining protein balance is augmented by maintenance of normal amino acid levels [10]. This emphasis on the ability of insulin levels to alter protein degradation while minimally effecting protein synthesis or fractional synthesis rate is substantiated by *in vivo* studies performed in adult rat heart muscle [12]. These studies also implicate degradation rather than synthesis as the primary factor effected by insulin and contradict earlier reports in which protein synthesis is increased by insulin infusion [15]. Also, in euglycemic animals, the effect of hemodynamic load and heart rate on protein turnover, have been shown to predominantly effect protein degradation as opposed to synthesis suggesting that this element of protein turnover may have a greater contribution to maintenance of protein content of the heart [16, 17].

Insulin may also influence fetal growth [18, 19] although the mechanisms by which this hormone modulates muscle growth and development remain to be elucidated. Johnson *et al.* [11] examined the effects of transuteral injection of insulin at day 19 of gestation on tissue protein turnover and nucleic acids. Using the flooding technique of assessing protein synthesis *in vivo*, [20] insulin infusions were associated with increased protein content and synthesis despite the fact that fractional synthesis and protein degradation were reportedly unchanged. While these data support the role of insulin as a growth factor in the developing heart it is unclear how increases in protein content were observed without a demonstrable decrease in protein degradation or increase in fractional synthesis rate. In a related study, the effect of streptozotocin-induced diabetes in pregnant female rats was examined in overall fetal protein synthesis and organ weights between 14 and 21 days of gestation [21]. While total fetal protein synthesis was depressed and protein degradation was elevated, heart weight of the fetus was unaffected by maternal diabetes (35 ± 0.9 mg) versus the control heart (34 ± 1.6 mg). It is important to note that the fetal heart, in contrast to the adult heart, may exhibit a protein synthetic response indicative of its maturational stage and may not be as sensitive to changes in insulin levels. It is also plausible that changes in total protein synthesis and degradation as described in this study do not adequately reflect the changes that occur in individual organ protein turnover, since the relative contribution of protein synthesis in the heart to total organism protein synthesis is not substantial.

Protein synthesis may also be affected by noncarbohydrate substrates in conjunction with insulin levels [22]. Earlier studies in the isolated rat heart suggest that insulin maintains protein and ribosomal synthesis [23]. However, when hearts from diabetic animals were perfused without insulin but in the presence of palmitate, normal protein synthetic rates were also observed [24]. Hearts from diabetic rats did display decreased uptake of phenylalanine when perfused for 3 hours with glucose in the absence of insulin and these differences were attributed to a block in peptide chain initiation. The blockage of peptide chain initiation was reversed in the diabetic heart after perfusion with palmitate suggesting that fatty acids may play a synergistic role in peptide chain initiation and protein synthesis.

The effects of diabetes on protein synthesis

The studies cited above suggest that while insulin plays an important role in maintaining protein synthesis and mass where glucose is the predominant substrate, the direct effect of insulin on synthetic rate of both the *in vivo* and *in vitro* perfused heart is not as clearly defined. In streptozotocin- or alloxan-diabetic rats the changes seen in protein synthesis appear to be more related to the duration of insulin deprivation rather than simply the absence of this hormone [25]. The reduction in the rate of protein synthesis has been attributed to a decrease in ribosomal concentration which is correlated with the duration of diabetes [25]. When perfused hearts from alloxan-diabetic animals were examined after 10 days of diabetes, the levels of cardiac protein synthesis, measured by phenylalanine incorporation, were depressed [26]. There was also a 22% reduction in cardiac RNA content suggesting that the inhibition in protein synthesis could be partly due to a reduced synthetic capacity while the remaining decrement in synthesis was attributed to a 10-15% reduction in efficiency. The mechanism postulated for the increased degradation in RNA may be accumulation of ribosomal subunits that are more vulnerable to degradation secondary to the decrease in protein synthesis [27]. Despite the decrease in RNA content observed in the diabetic heart, overall cardiac protein degradation was unchanged compared to control hearts.

Pain *et al.* [28] assessed the effect of streptozotocin-induced diabetes in rats at different times (4 and 56 days) after withdrawal of insulin therapy. Protein synthesis decreased in both skeletal and cardiac muscle and was attributed primarily to decreases in ribosomal concentration, particularly in the heart and in slow-twitch skeletal muscle. This fall in ribosome concentration was associated entirely with the decrease in protein synthesis while the efficiency was unchanged. In contrast, Garlick *et al.* [15] found that rates of protein degradation were elevated in diabetic hearts. However, these values were indirectly derived from protein synthesis and muscle protein content measured over time in

89

diabetic animals and not from direct measurements of protein degradation.

Using a large bolus injection of ^{3}H-phenylalanine, Ashford and Pain, [29] measured cardiac protein synthesis in acute diabetic animals (2nd and 4th day following insulin withdrawal). The rate of ribosomal synthesis was also assessed using a double tracer infusion technique [20]. Initially ^{14}C-leucine was infused followed by ^{3}H-leucine while the synthesis rate of ribosomes relative to total protein was assessed. Two days after withdrawal of insulin there was a substantial decrease in ribosomal content caused by a decrease in ribosomal synthesis and an elevation in degradation. By four days, both synthesis and degradation were depressed resulting in little change in ribosome content. Total tissue protein also decreased at 2 and 4 days and was due mainly to a decrease in synthesis with minimal changes in degradation. While these results suggest that diabetes affects protein synthesis by modulating ribosome synthesis and degradation, the data need to be interpreted with some caution since the rate of ribosomal and total cardiac protein synthesis were calculated over a 10 min interval and extrapolated to a 24-hour period, while the rate of degradation was indirectly calculated from changes in ribosome and protein content over a 24-48 hour period. Nevertheless, the large differences observed in ribosomal content of the diabetic compared to control heart coupled with alterations in ribosomal synthesis and degradation suggest that this step in protein synthesis plays an important role in altering overall cardiac protein synthesis with diabetes.

In a companion study, Ashford and Pain [30] examined synthesis and degradation of ribosomes and cardiac tissue protein during the acute phase of response to the replacement of insulin therapy to diabetic rats. Their findings are consistent with their earlier work in that total cardiac protein synthesis was modestly increased following insulin replacement in diabetic rats whereas ribosomal degradation was markedly reduced and synthesis was increased. The authors concluded that the low total protein degradation rates in the early phase of insulin therapy play an important role in permitting the accelerated rate of muscle growth during recovery. This was reflected in the increased synthesis and decreased degradation of ribosomes.

The acute protein synthetic response to insulin is recapitulated in the atrophied heart in response to increase heart rate. This may reflect the potential for cardiac muscle to alter protein degradation in an early phase of recovery from a physiologic insult. For example, in intact hearts exposed to reduced hemodynamic load and denervation, increased heart rate resulted in elevated protein synthesis as measured by the continuous infusion method. This was not attributed to increased fractional synthetic rate but to decreased protein degradation since left ventricular total protein content was increased without significant changes in fractional synthesis rates. It is apparent from our studies that protein degradation, was accelerated in these hearts, and increased heart rate attenuated this increased degradation [16,17]. Tolnai and Korecky have reported that lysosomal hydrolases, cathepsin D, glucosaminidase, and p-nitrophenolphosphatase are elevated in the atrophied heart [31]. It is plausible that in our model of reduced hemodynamic load and denervation, increased hydrolase activity may contribute to the cardiac atrophy observed and that increased heart rate may alter the activity of these enzymes. Whether insulin deficiency may also effect cardiac protein turnover by modulating hydrolase activity is unknown.

Along with the observed changes in ribosomal RNA, protein synthesis is also altered by changes in the initiation and elongation of the peptide chain [32,33]. The effect of alloxan-induced diabetes on eukaryotic initiation factor-2B (IF-2B) activity was assessed in skeletal and cardiac muscle [32]. The first step in peptide chain initiation is formation of a complex arising from IF-2, GTP, and methionyl-tRNA. The rate of peptide chain initiation can be regulated by this reaction which is dependent on IF-2B, an exchange factor required for recycling IF-2. Initiation factor-2B exchange is inhibited in fast-twitch skeletal muscle of diabetic rats [34,35], whereas in cardiac muscle it is unchanged. Consistent with previously published findings, these investigators demonstrated that insulin may control the IF-2B-mediated exchange of IF-2 bound GDP for GTP in peptide-chain initiation by altering phosphorylation of casein kinase II, an enzyme which is decreased during the inhibition of IF-2B in fast-twitch skeletal muscle of diabetic animals. In contrast, IF-2B levels in cardiac and slow-twitch skeletal muscle are unaffected by diabetes and suggest that

91

the ability of these muscles to utilize free fatty acids as substrate for energy may play a protective role in decreased synthesis associated with the disease.

In contrast to the ability of cardiac muscle to sustain peptide-chain initiation in alloxan-induced diabetes, inhibiting elongation of the peptide chain may occur in the heart when the duration of insulin deficiency is increased [33]. In alloxan-induced diabetic rats, ribosomal content was reduced by 28% after 48 hours of insulin deficiency while both ribosomal content and translational efficiency (30%) were reduced in cardiac muscle when the duration of diabetes was increased to 72 hours. This also resulted in a 37% reduction in peptide-chain elongation. Treatment with insulin for 3 days was sufficient to reverse the effects on protein synthesis, ribosomal content and translational efficiency. Coincident with the decrease in translation efficiency was a 66% decrease in elongation factor-2 (EF-2) which was also reversed with insulin therapy. These data suggest that EF-2 plays a regulatory role in maintaining protein synthesis by altering elongation/termination of the peptide chain.

Contractile protein abnormalities in diabetes

Insulin deficient diabetes elicits alterations in contractile protein synthesis and marked changes in cardiac function which are hallmarks of the diabetic heart [36,37]. Numerous investigators have conducted mechanical, ultrastructural and biochemical studies in different animal models demonstrating that diabetes influences myocardial contractility and changes in cardiac energetics [36, 38-42]. Penpargkul *et al.* [43] explored the effects of streptozotocin-induced diabetes on cardiac performance and metabolism indicating an abnormal myocardial function in rats. In a study of left ventricular function after chronic insulin treatment in diabetic rats, complete reversal of streptozotocin-induced cardiomyopathy suggested that this condition was due to insulin deficiency and not due to a primary cardiotoxic effect of streptozotocin [44]. We and others also demonstrated altered papillary muscle mechanics and changes in contractile proteins in the alloxan-induced diabetic rabbit model [45,46]. Diminished velocity of shortening, an increased duration of isometric contraction-relaxation and contractile proteins were the prominent abnormalities observed that could be reversed by insulin therapy [42]. Pierce and Dhalla have described a depressed cardiac myofibrillar adenosine triphosphatase activity (ATPase) in diabetic rats, which is correlated with the above changes in contractile dysfunction [47]. Others have demonstrated that ß-myosin heavy chain, the isoform of cardiac myosin correlated with decreased ATPase activity and shortening velocity, is the predominant isoform of myosin in chronic diabetes and that contractile proteins other than myosin may be altered in the diabetic heart [39,41].

Along with the direct effects of insulin withdrawal and replacement on isomyosin expression and cardiac function, related work from our laboratory demonstrates that isomyosin expression, total cardiac protein synthesis and fractional synthesis rates are directly altered by chronic catecholamine and angiotensin II administration, which may also be indirectly influenced by hypo- or hyperinsulinemia. In heterotopically transplanted hearts exposed to a reduced hemodynamic load, decreased α-myosin heavy chain expression was directly correlated with a loss of cardiac protein. When these hearts were exposed to chronic ß-adrenergic stimulation, the decrease in α-myosin heavy chain was attenuated independent of changes in protein synthesis whereas exposure to angiotensin II altered protein synthesis but not isomyosin expression [48,49]. These studies suggest that insulin, another endogenous hormone, may also contribute to changes in isomyosin expression but that its effect on cardiac protein turnover may be dissociated from these qualitative changes in cardiac muscle protein. In vertebrate striated muscle, regulatory components of the thin filaments troponin and tropomyosin are responsible, in part, for transducing the effect of free calcium in contractile protein activation and for inhibiting this activity when calcium is absent [50]. Enzymatic data based on hybridization studies from our laboratory suggest that besides the shift of α- to ß-isomyosin and depressed myosin ATPase, troponin-tropomyosin may play a seminal role in the regulation of the actomyosin system in diabetic cardiomyopathy [51].

Summary

While protein turnover in fast-twitch skeletal muscle of diabetic animals is primarily altered by an increase in degradation and is heavily dependent on availability of glucose, cardiac muscle protein turnover in diabetes is effected by changes in protein synthesis and is less dependent on glucose as a substrate for maintaining muscle mass similar to slow-twitch skeletal muscle. It is unclear whether changes in total cardiac protein turnover in the diabetic animal actually reflect changes in synthesis or degradation of individual contractile proteins. Previous data suggest that specific myosin heavy chain protein expression is altered in diabetes and that these modifications of the contractile machinery and the resulting decrement in cardiac function can be attributed directly to diabetes. Direct measurements of myosin heavy chain protein synthesis and synthesis of the regulatory proteins in the diabetic heart and isolated cardiac tissue will aid in elucidating the intracellular mechanisms responsible for the changes in protein expression which accompany this disease process.

References

1. Pain VM and Garlick PJ. Effect of streptozotocin diabetes and insulin treatment on the rate of protein synthesis in tissues of the rat in vivo. *J. Biol. Chem.* **261**: 4066-4070, 1974.

2. Gelfand RA and Barrett EJ. Effects of physiologic hyperinsulinemia on skeletal muscle protein synthesis and breakdown in man. *J. Clin. Invest.* **80**: 1-6, 1987.

3. Evans CD, Schreiber SS, Oratz M and Rothschild MA. Relative synthesis of cardiac contractile proteins. Evidence for synthesis from the same precursor pool. *Biochem. J.* **194**: 673-675, 1981.

4. Martin AF. Turnover of cardiac troponin subunits. *J. Biol. Chem.* **256**: 964-968, 1981.

5. Zak R, Martin AF, Prior G and Rabinowitz M. Comparison of turnover of several myofibrillar proteins and critical

evaluation of the double isotope method. *J. Biol. Chem.* **252**: 3430-3435, 1977.

6. Everett AW and Zak R. Problems and interpretations of techniques used in studies of protein turnover, in Wildenthal (ed): *Degradative processes in heart and skeletal muscle.* Elsevier/North Holland Biomedical Press, pp 31-47, 1980.

7. Morgan HE, Jefferson LS, Wolpert EB and Rannels DE. Regulation of protein synthesis in heart muscle. II. Effect of amino acid levels and insulin on ribosomal aggregation. *J. Biol. Chem.* **246**: 2163-2170, 1971.

8. Rannels DE, Kao R and Morgan HE. Effect of insulin on protein turnover in heart muscle. *J. Biol. Chem.* **250**: 1694-1701, 1975.

9. Flaim KE, Kochel PJ, Kira Y, Kobayashi K, Fossel ET, Jefferson LS and Morgan HE. Insulin effects on protein synthesis are independent of glucose and energy metabolism. *Am. J. Physiol.* **245**: C133-C143, 1983

10. Young LH and Dahl DM. Physiological hyperinsulinemia inhibits myocardial protein degradation in vivo in the canine heart. *Circ. Res.* **71**: 393-400, 1992.

11. Johnson JD, Dunham T, Wogenrich FJ, Greenberg RE, Loftfield RB and Skipper BJ. Fetal hyperinsulinemia and protein turnover in fetal rat tissues. *Diabetes* **39**: 541-548, 1990.

12. McNulty PH, Young LH and Barrett EJ. Response of rat heart and skeletal muscle protein in vivo to insulin and amino acid infusion. *Am. J. Physiol.* **264**: E958-965, 1993.

13. Young LH and Stirewalt WS. Effect of insulin on rat heart and skeletal muscle phenylalanyl-tRNA labeling and protein synthesis in vivo. *Am. J. Physiol.* **267**: E337-342, 1994.

14. Revkin JH, Young LH, Stirewalt WS, Dahl DM, Gelfand RA, Zaret BL and Barrett EJ. In vivo measurement of myocardial protein turnover using an indicator dilution technique. *Circ. Res.* **67**: 902-912, 1990.

15. Garlick PJ, Fern M and Preedy VR. The effect of insulin infusion and food intake on muscle protein synthesis in post absorptive rats. *Biochem. J.* **210**: 669-676, 1983.

16. Geenen DL, Malhotra A, Buttrick PM and Scheuer J. Increased heart rate prevents the isomyosin shift after cardiac transplantation in the rat. *Circ. Res.* **70**: 554-558, 1992.

17. Geenen DL, Malhotra A, Buttrick PM and Scheuer J. Ventricular pacing attenuates but does not reverse cardiac atrophy and an isomyosin shift in the rat heart. *Am. J. Physiol.* **267**: H2149-H2154, 1994.

18. Picon L. Effect of insulin on growth and biochemical composition of the rat fetus. *Endocrinology* **81**: 1419-1421, 1967.

19. Susa JB, McCormick KL, Widness JA, Singer DB, Oh W, Adamsons K and Schwartz R. Chronic hyperinsulinemia in the fetal rhesus monkey: effects on fetal growth and composition. *Diabetes* **28**: 1058-1063, 1979.

20. Garlick PJ, McNurlan MA and Preedy VR. A rapid and convenient technique for measuring the rate of protein synthesis in tissues by injection of ^{3}H-phenylalanine. *Biochem. J.* **192**: 719-723, 1980.

21. Canavan JP and Goldspink DF. Maternal diabetes in rats. II. Effects on fetal growth and protein turnover. *Diabetes* **37**: 1671-1617, 1988.

22. Rannels DE, Hjalmarson AC and Morgan HE. Effects of noncarbohydrate substrates on protein synthesis in muscle. *Am. J. Physiol.* **226**: 528-539, 1974.

23. Neely JR, Bowman RH and Morgan HE. Effects of ventricular pressure development and palmitate on glucose transport. *Am. J. Physiol.* **216**: 804-811, 1969.

24. Rannels DE, Jefferson LS, Hjalmarson AC, Wolpert EB and Morgan HE. Maintenance of protein synthesis in hearts of diabetic animals. *Biochem. Biophys. Res. Comm.* **40**: 1110-1116, 1970.

25. Wool IG, Rampersad OR and Moyer AN. Effect of insulin and diabetes on protein synthesis by ribosomes from heart muscle. Significance for theories of the hormone's mechanism of action. *Am. J. Med.* **40**: 716-723, 1966.

26. Williams IH, Chua BHL, Sahms RH, Siehl D and Morgan HE. Effects of diabetes on protein turnover in cardiac muscle. *Am. J. Physiol.* **239**: E178-E185, 1980.

27. Millward DJ, Garlick PJ, James WPT, Nnanyelugo DO and Ryatt JS. Relationship between protein synthesis and RNA content in skeletal muscle. *Nature* **241**:204-205, 1973.

28. Pain VM, Albertse EC and Garlick PJ. Protein metabolism in skeletal muscle, diaphragm, and heart of diabetic rats. *Am. J. Physiol.* **245**: E604-E610, 1983.

29. Ashford AJ and Pain VM. Effect of diabetes on the rates of synthesis and degradation of ribosomes in rat muscle and liver in vivo. *J. Biol. Chem.* **261**: 4059-4065, 1986.

30. Ashford AJ and Pain VM. Insulin stimulation of growth in diabetic rats. Synthesis and degradation of ribosomes and total tissue protein in skeletal muscle and heart. *J. Biol. Chem.* **261**: 4066-4070, 1986.

31. Tolnai S and Korecky B. Lysosomal hydrolases in the heterotopically isotransplanted heart undergoing atrophy. *J. Mol. Cell. Cardiol.* **12**: 869-890, 1980.

32. Karinch AM, Kimball SR, Vary TC and Jefferson LS. Regulation of eukaryotic initiation factor-2B activity in muscle of diabetic rats. *Am. J. Physiol.* **264**: E101-E108, 1993.

33. Vary TC, Nairn A and Lynch CJ. Role of elongation factor 2 in regulating peptide-chain elongation in the heart. *Am. J. Physiol.* **266**: E628-E634, 1994.

34. Jeffrey IW, Kelly FJ, Duncan R, Hershey JWB and Pain VM. Effect of starvation and diabetes on the activity of the eukaryotic initiation factor eIF-2 in rat skeletal muscle. *Biochimie* **72**: 751-757, 1990.

35. Kimball SR and Jefferson LS. Effect of diabetes on guanine nucleotide exchange factor activity in skeletal muscle and heart. *Biochem. Biophys. Res. Comm.* **156**: 706-711, 1988.

36. Fein FS, Kornstein LB, Strobeck JE, Capasso JM and Sonnenblick EH. Altered myocardial mechanics in diabetic rats. *Circ. Res.* **47**: 922-933, 1980.

37. Regan TJ, Lyons MM, Ahmed SS, Levinson GE, Oldewurtel HA, Ahmed MR and Haider B. Evidence for cardiomyopathy in familial diabetes mellitus. *J. Clin. Invest.* **60**: 885-899, 1977.

38. Takeda N, Nakamura I, Hatanaka T, Ohkubo T and Nagano M. Myocardial mechanical and myosin isoenzyme alterations in streptozotocin-diabetic rats. *Japan Heart J.* **29**: 455-463, 1988.

39. Malhotra A, Penpargkul S, Fein FS, Sonnenblick EH and Scheuer J. The effect of streptozotocin induced diabetes in rats on cardiac contractile proteins. *Circ. Res.* **49**: 1243-1250, 1981.

40. Fein FS, Cho S, Malhotra A, Akella J, Vanhoeven KH, Sonnenblick EH and Factor SM. Beneficial effects of diltiazem on the natural history of hypertensive-diabetic cardiomyopathy in rats. *J. Am. Coll. Cardiol.* **18**: 1406-1417, 1991.

41. Malhotra A, Fein FS and Lopez MC. Regulatory proteins (Troponin-Tropomyosin) in diabetic cardiomyopathy. *Biophys. J.* **59**: 587a, 1991.

42. Fein FS, Strobeck JE, Malhotra A, Scheuer J and Sonnenblick EH. Reversibility of diabetic cardiomyopathy with insulin in rats. *Circ. Res.* **49**: 1251-1261, 1981.

43. Penpargkul S, Schaible T, Yipintsoi T and Scheuer J. The effects of diabetes on performance and metabolism of rat hearts. *Circ. Res.* **49**:9 11-921, 1980.

44. Schaible TF, Malhotra A, Bauman WA and Scheuer J. Left ventricular function after chronic insulin treatment in diabetic and normal rats. *J. Mol. Cell. Cardiol.* **15**: 445-458, 1983.

45. Fein FS, Miller-Green B and Sonnenblick EH. Altered myocardial mechanics in diabetic rabbits. *Am. J. Physiol.* **248**: H729-H736, 1985.

46. Pollack PS, Malhotra A, Fein FS and Scheuer J. Effects of diabetes on cardiac contractile proteins in rabbits and reversal with insulin. *Am. J. Physiol.* **251**: H448-H454, 1986.

47. Pierce GN and Dhalla NS. Cardiac myofibrillar ATPase activity in diabetic rats. *J. Mol. Cell. Cardiol.* **13**: 1063-1069, 1981.

48. Geenen DL, Malhotra A, Scheuer J and Buttrick PM. Repeated catecholamine surges alter cardiac isomyosin distribution but not protein synthesis in the rat heart. *Am. J. Physiol.* (In Review)

49. Geenen DL, Malhotra A and Scheuer J. Angiotensin II increases cardiac protein synthesis in adult rat heart. *Am. J. Physiol.* **265**: H238-H243, 1993.

50. Ebashi S, Nonomura Y, Kohama K, Kitazawa T and Mikawa T. Regulation of muscle contraction by Ca ion. *Mol. Biol. Biochem. Biophys.* **32**:183-194, 1980.

51. Malhotra A, Lopez C and Nakouzi A. Troponin subunits contribute to altered myosin ATPase activity in diabetic cardiomyopathy. *Mol. Cell. Biochem. (In Press)* 1995.

CHAPTER 6

Remodelling of Subcellular Organelles During the Development of Diabetic Cardiomyopathy

Naranjan S. Dhalla
Leonard S. Golfman
Vijayan Elimban
Nobuakira Takeda

Introduction

In view of the fact that cardiac contractile force development is a cellular event, much data have accumulated in the literature to support a close association between changes in the intracellular concentration of calcium and the status of heart function. Accordingly, mechanisms which regulate calcium homeostasis in the cell and components which interact with calcium are considered important determinants of the heart function. Several organelles such as the sarcolemmal membrane, the sarcoplasmic reticulum (SR), the mitochondria, and the contractile proteins in the myocardial cell are involved in the control of intracellular calcium, contractile force generation and relaxation in the heart. Since these organelles are important for the viability of the healthy myocardium, it is reasonable to assume that a lesion in one or more of these organelles may be associated with a depression of cardiac function commonly observed in chronic diabetes. The possibility that functional abnormalities associated with diabetes mellitus may result from significant remodelling of various organelles has been addressed by a number of laboratories. Alterations in different subcellular organelles have been identified and extensive investigations have been carried out to characterize the nature of such abnormalities in diabetic heart. In this chapter, a discussion concerning the remodelling of the contractile proteins, sarcolemma, mitochondria, and SR in cardiac tissue from diabetic animals is presented. An attempt has been made to understand how these changes may relate to the observed depression in force generation in the diabetic myocardium.

Contractile protein changes

The final reaction in the sequence of subcellular events leading to cardiac contraction lies at the level of contractile proteins. Calcium binding to troponin C protein allows myosin to interact with the actin through a conformational change [1]. In this process, adenosine triphosphate (ATP) is hydrolyzed to adenosine diphosphate (ADP) and inorganic phosphate (Pi) by the enzyme adenosine triphosphatase (ATPase), which is located on the head region of the myosin molecule [2]. The observation that the myofibrillar ATPase activity is related to cardiac contractile force development [3] has allowed investigators to utilize this biochemical marker of contractile protein function to gain information regarding cardiac performance. It is possible to separate contractile proteins by various means into distinct preparations of varying purity [2]. Several preparations of contractile proteins are presently examined routinely by many laboratories but four fractions have achieved widespread use: myofibrils, actomyosin, myosin, and heavy meromyosin. The myofibrillar preparation contains a more complete complement of contractile proteins and, therefore, may represent a closer approximation of the actual physiological setting [2]. However, many experiments require a purer preparation of contractile proteins to avoid possible errors in interpretation of results. The myosin or heavy meromyosin preparations represent the contractile proteins as a single protein. Each "preparation" has its own advantages and disadvantages [2] and such considerations will thus limit the value of the conclusions which are obtained from extensive investigations.

Purified myofibrillar fractions, isolated from hearts of streptozotocin (STZ)-induced diabetic rats, showed depressed Ca^{2+}-stimulated ATPase activities in comparison to control [4-6]. This defect was found to be closely associated with the hyperglycemic status of diabetic animals. If this condition was corrected by chronic insulin administration, Ca^{2+}-stimulated ATPase activity returned to normal [4,5]. The depression in Ca^{2+}-stimulated ATPase activity of cardiac myofibrils from diabetic animals was observed over a full range of physiologically relevant calcium concentrations [4,7]. Myofibrillar Mg^{2+}-dependent ATPase activity in diabetic animals also exhibited a similar loss in comparison to control preparations and this change was eliminated after chronic administration of insulin to diabetic animals [5]. Studies with alloxan diabetic rabbits [7,8] have also revealed a decrease in myofibrillar Ca^{2+}-stimulated ATPase activity with subsequent normalization upon insulin administration.

The mechanism responsible for the defect in myofibrillar ATPase activity has been difficult to identify but several possibilities have been put forward. Gross changes due to cross contamination in myofibrils were considered unlikely since sodium dodecyl sulfate (SDS) electrophoretic analysis of myofibrillar samples revealed no significant differences between control and diabetic preparations [9]. Phosphorylation of specific proteins in the myofibrillar fraction is known to influence myofibrillar Ca^{2+}-ATPase activity. However, this may not be responsible for the observed changes because similar levels of *in vitro* phosphorylation in both control and diabetic cardiac myofibrillar fractions were observed [9]. Certainly, it is not a direct effect of the decrease in insulin levels in the circulation of diabetic animals since insulin had no action on myofibrillar function [9]. In one study the myofibrillar fraction from diabetic rat heart was found to exhibit a different reactivity to sulfhydryl group modifiers in comparison to the control [5]; such an alteration supports the contention that conformational changes near the active site of ATPase exist in diabetic myofibrils and may be an important factor in the observed enzymatic changes [4,5]. Nonetheless, in view of the fact that the significance of myofibrillar Ca^{2+}-stimulated ATPase activity lies in its close relationship with force generation [10], the depression in myofibrillar ATPase activity in hearts from diabetic animals may account for the contractile dysfunction. Dillman [11] was the first to report detailed evidence of contractile protein defects in the heart during diabetes mellitus. Ca^{2+}-activated ATPase activities of actomyosin and myosin Ca^{2+}-ATPase were observed to be significantly depressed in hearts from diabetic animals. These results were confirmed by other investigators [12-14].

Table 6.1 **Myofibrillar Ca^{2+}-stimulated ATPase and myosin Ca^{2+}-ATPase activities in control, diabetic and verapamil-treated diabetic rats.**

	Control	Diabetic	Verapamil-treated Diabetic
Myofibrillar Ca^{2+}-stimulated ATPase (nmol Pi/mg/min)	148±7.4	95±6.3*	141±15.4#
Myosin Ca^{2+}-ATPase (nmol P_i/mg/ min)	298±10.2	86±7.5*	195±17.1#

*Each value is a mean ± S.E. of 6 to 8 experiments. * = P < 0.05 (Diabetic vs. Control); # = P < 0.05 (Treated vs. Untreated Diabetic). The results described here are taken from our study reported previously [6]. Diabetes was induced by a single injection of streptozotocin in the femoral vein (65 mg/kg). For the verapamil-treated diabetic group, the animals one day after the induction of diabetes were injected 8 mg/kg verapamil (subcutaneously in two doses - one at 9:00 a.m. and the other at 5:00 p.m. daily) for a period of 8 weeks. The diabetic group received saline injections throughout the 8 week period.*

The existence of changes in cardiac myosin K^+-EDTA ATPase activity in diabetic animals is controversial but caloric considerations were found not to be a factor for the observed depression in myosin Ca^{2+}-ATPase activity [15]. The alterations in myosin ATPase activity were dependent upon the duration of the diabetic condition and were present irrespective of the sex of the animal. It was also shown that the accompanying hypothyroid status of diabetic animals was not a primary factor responsible for the depression in myosin Ca^{2+}-ATPase activity [14-16]. Nonetheless, diabetes-induced depression in both myosin Ca^{2+}-ATPase and myofibrillar Ca^{2+}-stimulated ATPase activities were prevented upon treating the diabetic animals with a calcium-antagonist, verapamil (Table 6.1); this indicated that the occurrence of intracellular calcium overload in diabetic heart may be involved in inducing myofibrillar alterations.

Pyrophosphate gel electrophoresis of myosin isoenzyme components from control and diabetic rat hearts revealed significant mobility changes [11]. The myosin V_1, or high mobility component, was predominant whereas myosin V_3, the lowest mobility myosin component, existed in relatively small amounts in control rat heart. This pattern was reversed, however, in the myosin samples prepared from diabetic rat hearts; V_3 fraction was the predominant component whereas the V_1 component was very low in content. The observed changes in the myosin isoenzyme distribution in experimental preparations could be reversed if the diabetic animals were treated with insulin [11,15], verapamil [6] and different metabolic and lipid lowering interventions [17,18]. It should be noted that a predominance of the V_1 component of myosin has been correlated with high activity of myosin Ca^{2+}-ATPase enzyme and maximal shortening velocity in cardiac muscle preparations [19,20]. Conversely, a predominance of the myosin V_3 component has been associated with lower myosin Ca^{2+}-ATPase activity and reduced shortening velocity in cardiac muscle preparations. Thus the depression in myosin Ca^{2+}-ATPase activity in diabetic rat heart may be a result of the observed change in isoenzyme distribution. Since different isoenzymic forms of myosin are under genetic control [21], it would appear that changes in contractile proteins during the development of diabetic cardiomyopathy may be at the level of gene expression. Work in this area has confirmed that a reduction in the translational activity of specific messenger ribonucleic acids for heavy chain myosin is evident in diabetic rat hearts [22].

Sarcoplasmic reticulum changes

One of the main functions of the sarcoplasmic reticulum (SR) membrane system is to release calcium from its stores into the cytoplasm to support contraction and to take up calcium into its cisternae from the cytoplasm to effect relaxation. The relative contribution of the SR to the calcium transient appears to exist with respect to species as rat myocardium receives the largest contribution and rabbit heart the least [23]. The SR network borders the myofibrillar contractile apparatus as well as the sarcolemma and the T-tubule system. The energy-dependent calcium uptake process of the SR depends on the function of Ca^{2+}-stimulated ATPase which is believed to represent 50%-90% of the total protein content of the SR [24]. The calcium affinity (K_m of 0.5 μmol/L) and V_{max} of Ca^{2+}-stimulated ATPase are sufficiently high to support the concept that the activity of this enzyme is the primary determinant of the rate of fall of the calcium transient [25] in the cardiac muscle. Experimentally, it has been convenient to measure ATP-dependent calcium uptake in the absence or presence of a precipitating anion, like oxalate. Oxalate will precipitate free calcium which accumulates in the SR membrane vesicle during calcium transport; this will stabilize the intravesicular free Ca^{2+}-binding because the high intravesicular free calcium level is considered to act as a feedback regulator of the SR Ca^{2+}-pump and inhibit its activity. Quantitation of calcium uptake is not the only measure of SR Ca^{2+}-pump function, ATP hydrolysis by the Ca^{2+}-pump protein is also monitored to express the Ca^{2+}-stimulated ATPase activity [25]. Since cardiac muscle from diabetic animals exhibits a slower rate of relaxation than that of controls [26], it has been hypothesized that an abnormality in the removal of Ca^{2+} from the cytoplasm after contraction may be present in the diabetic heart. Investigators from New York [27] were first to identify a depression in the Ca^{2+}-accumulating capacity of SR membrane vesicles isolated from the hearts of diabetic animals. This observation was confirmed and the conclusions extended by several other investigators [6,28-30]. Not only is calcium uptake depressed in SR, studies have also shown a decrease in calcium binding [30] when examined as a function of calcium concentrations.

Affected SR calcium transport in the diabetic heart has been associated with concomitant defects in Ca^{2+}-stimulated ATPase activity [6,28,30]. The SR Mg^{2+}-ATPase activity in diabetic rat heart has also been shown to be depressed [27] or unaffected [30]. Nonetheless, results from different laboratories are consistent with the interpretation that a lesion in the SR calcium transport system is present in the myocardium from diabetic animals. This defect appears to be a direct result of the diabetes since it becomes evident under chronic conditions; the defect in SR calcium transport is gradual in onset, appearing 2 weeks after the diabetic condition [30]. Insulin treatment of diabetic animals was found to reverse the changes in Ca^{2+}-stimulated ATPase activity [30] and calcium uptake by the SR [29,30]. Although a direct action of insulin on SR calcium transport has been reported [31], it is not clear whether this effect actually plays any role in the defects observed in the insulin-deficient diabetic state.

It has been suggested that the hypothyroid state of the diabetic animals could be responsible for the defect in SR function. In this regard, it should be noted that hypothyroidism has been shown to cause a depression in cardiac SR calcium transport [32]. However, treatment of diabetic animals with thyroxine to restore circulating thyroid hormone levels did not abolish the defect in cardiac SR calcium uptake activity [30]. Thus, it was concluded that the hypothyroid state of the diabetic animals was not responsible for the lesion. Although some changes in lipid composition of the microsomal fraction were evident [30], these alterations were not dramatic and were thought to be unlikely to fully explain the membrane dysfunction. Furthermore, changes in the regulation of calcium transport by various phosphorylation mechanisms did not appear to occur as *in vitro* measurements of this parameter with cardiac SR membranes from diabetic animals did not reveal significant alterations [33].

It has been suggested that the accumulation of lipids in the myocardium which occurs during diabetes [34] may be involved in the defect in SR function. In particular, long-chain acylcarnitines like palmitoylcarnitine are known to accumulate in the hearts of diabetic animals [28,34] and such compounds have been shown to inhibit the function of SR [35,36]. Since the inhibition of control SR calcium transport by long-chain acylcarnitines was greater than that observed in diabetic preparations [28], it was suggested that some inhibition of SR function in the diabetic preparations may be due to high endogenous levels of these lipid moieties. However, all these parameters were normalized in diabetic animals by D,L-carnitine treatment but cardiac performance remained depressed [29]. This would suggest an important dissociation of SR function from cardiac function and imply that other factors besides lesions in the SR membrane system may be responsible for heart dysfunction in diabetic cardiomyopathy. However, this may be a premature conclusion because other investigators have demonstrated that treatment of diabetic animals with L-carnitine normalized cardiac performance [37] and carnitine treatment was found to prevent the diabetes-induced changes in the sarcoplasmic reticular Ca^{2+} pump system [38]. Treatment of diabetic animals with verapamil, which was shown to partially prevent changes in heart function [39], was also found to prevent depressions in SR Ca^{2+}-uptake and Ca^{2+}-stimulated ATPase activities (Table 6.2).

Table 6.2: Cardiac sarcoplasmic reticular Ca^{2+}-pump activities in control, diabetic and verapamil-treated diabetic rats.

	Control	Diabetic	Verapamil-treated Diabetic
Ca^{2+}-uptake (nmol Ca^{2+}/mg/ 5 min)	183±15	113±16*	210±12#
Ca^{2+}-stimulated ATPase (nmol Ca^{2+}/ mg/ 5 min)	0.89±0.08	0.52±0.05*	0.92±0.06#

*Each value is a mean ± S.E. of 4 to 6 experiments. * = P < 0.05 (Diabetic vs. Control); # = P < 0.05 (Treated vs. Untreated Diabetic). The results described here are taken from our study reported previously [6]. The induction of diabetes and verapamil treatment are the same as those in Table 6.1.*

In addition, recent studies by Katagiri et al. [40] with STZ rats demonstrated SR depression of Ca^{2+}-ATPase activity as early as one week before the appearance of fine ultrastructural alterations. Although depressed SR calcium transport activity in diabetic heart was considered to be due to a depression in the gene expression activity [41], no changes in the mRNA level for SR Ca^{2+}-pump [22,42] or SR Ca^{2+}-pump protein content [42] were observed in diabetic heart.

Mitochondrial changes

Since mitochondria have the capacity to accumulate large amounts of calcium and occupy a large volume of the myocardial cell, it was assumed that these organelles participate in regulating the intracellular concentration of calcium. However, this hypothesis was discounted because of two experimental observations. First, calcium uptake by the mitochondria was too slow to support beat to beat cardiac contraction and relaxation, and second, the affinity of mitochondria for calcium was far too low for mitochondrial calcium transport to be active at the micromolar concentrations of calcium, which are available during the excitation-contraction and relaxation processes in the heart [43]. The current view of calcium accumulation by mitochondria in the heart is that it may act as a sink for calcium under pathological conditions [44-46]. When calcium entry into the heart is excessive, cytoplasmic calcium concentrations rise and when this rise is too high, mitochondria will begin to accumulate calcium in an effort to prevent the occurrence of intracellular calcium overload. If the calcium in the cytoplasm is not controlled, the heart will lose its ability to relax, arrhythmias can develop, and lysosomal enzymes may be released which can be destructive to the myocardial cell [46,47]. Thus, mitochondria can be seen to act as an important buffering component of the cytoplasmic calcium levels in the diabetic heart. It has been hypothesized that chronic diabetes could influence mitochondrial performance and this dysfunction may be related to the diabetic cardiomyopathy, since alterations in mitochondrial morphology had been well documented [48,49].

Much work has been directed to an examination of oxidative metabolism in mitochondria from hearts of diabetic animals. It was Goranson and Erulkar [50] who first suggested the presence of a defect in mitochondrial oxidative phosphorylative activity in the heart during acute diabetes [51-54]. Phosphorylation of creatine in heart homogenates in the presence of succinate or malate was found to be depressed in alloxan-diabetic rats. A decreased synthesis of ATP and ADP in the presence of glucose, fructose and lactate was observed in heart homogenates from diabetic rats [52,53,55] 24 to 48 hours after alloxan injection. Chen and Ianuzzo [56] also described a decrease in cardiac succinate dehydrogenase activity during diabetes. Significant reductions in mitochondrial oxygen consumption and respiratory control index values were demonstrated in alloxan-diabetic hearts [53]. Subsequent investigations have documented significant defects in the respiratory capacity of mitochondria isolated from hearts of genetically diabetic as well as streptozotocin-diabetic rats [57-59]. Pierce and Dhalla [59] reported that mitochondria isolated from ventricular tissue by differential centrifugation from 8-week streptozotocin-induced diabetic rats had depressed state 3 respiration, oxidative phosphorylation rate, respiratory control index and depressed magnesium-dependent activities. These changes were partially reversed upon 2 weeks of insulin and fully reversible after 4 weeks of insulin therapy. State 4 respiration was normal during diabetes [57,59]. Overall, the depression in mitochondrial oxidative phosphorylation has been shown to become more severe as the duration of the diabetes lengthens and can be normalized by daily insulin treatment of diabetic animals.

Many investigators have reported a significant depression in high-energy phosphate content in hearts from diabetic animals [39,60-65] with depressed ATP synthesis rate [66,67]. In addition, phosphocreatine metabolism was abnormal in the heart during diabetes [63]. Since the creatine kinase (CK) isoenzymes, phosphocreatine, ATP and ADP (the phosphocreatine energy shuttle) play an important role in the process of energy production and utilization in cardiac muscle [68,69], an impairment of the system can be seen to result in deterioration of contractile function [67]. Savabi and Kirsch [68] reported a reduction in various CK isoenzymes, high-energy phosphates and mitochondrial oxidative phosphorylation in streptozotocin-diabetic rat hearts. These changes reached their maximum level after 4 weeks of diabetes and stayed constant thereafter. All of these diabetic related alterations were reversible by 4 weeks of insulin treatment. Other investigators [70] also showed that diabetes mellitus in the streptozotocin-diabetic rat resulted in a reduction of total CK activity and a redistribution of CK isoenzymes in the heart. Furthermore, a decrease in CK mRNA was associated with the observed decrease in CK activity; chronic insulin administration reversed these changes.

In addition to some of the defects observed in mitochondrial respiratory activity and phosphocreatine energy shuttle, mitochondrial calcium uptake capacity has been shown to be significantly depressed in hearts from diabetic animals in comparison to control preparations [59]. This depression was directly attributable to the diabetic condition since the defect was reversible by insulin administration to the diabetic animals. The depression in mitochondrial calcium uptake activity was not seen at low concentrations of calcium and was not associated with any change in calcium binding activity. Only high calcium concentrations revealed a lesion in the mitochondrial calcium uptake capacity in the diabetic preparations. The results with calcium transport by mitochondria from diabetic animals may be interpreted to suggest a defect in the calcium-accumulating capacity by these organelles and indicate that the diabetic mitochondria may have been unable to maintain large calcium concentration gradients across their membranes. It should be pointed out that previous studies from various laboratories showing derangements in mitochondrial respiration and calcium uptake in the diabetic heart were carried out by using isolated subcellular fractions, and represent data pooled from a mixed population of cells. Furthermore, most reports indicated that impairments in function of mitochondria were detectable 4 weeks or longer after the streptozotocin injection [59]. Some of the results showing remodelling of mitochondria at late stages of diabetes and the reversibility of mitochondrial changes by insulin are given in Table 6.3.

In a recent study by Tanaka *et al.* [71], calcium uptake by mitochondria, measured *in situ* in permeabilized cardiomyocytes of STZ-diabetic rats, was significantly decreased compared to that of control rats, regardless of the extramitochondrial (cytosolic) calcium concentration. Impairments were also observed in myocyte respiration and mitochondrial membrane potential. These mitochondrial dysfunctions were observed as early as 3 weeks after streptozotocin administration and were reversible by insulin treatment. The exact role of changes in mitochondrial calcium uptake in diabetic heart is not clear because a disturbance in calcium homeostasis of the heart cell was indicated by a decreased content of rapidly exchangeable $^{45}Ca^{2+}$ of the myocyte [71]. Since it is believed that the latter consists predominantly of calcium in the SR [72,73], the possibility that defects in mitochondrial calcium transport may be secondary to impairments in SR Ca^{2+}-pump activity in the diabetic heart cannot be ignored.

Table 6.3: Cardiac mitochondrial alterations in control, diabetic and insulin-treated diabetic rats

	Control	Diabetic	Insulin-treated diabetic
Ca^{2+}-uptake (nmol Ca^{2+}/mg/ 5 min)	124±3.8	98±2.7*	122±4.1
Mg^{2+}-ATPase activity (μmol P_i/mg/5 min)	8.2±0.6	5.7±0.3*	7.0±0.5
ADP/O ratio	2.92±0.20	2.48±0.25	2.87±0.15
Oxidative phosphorylation rate (nmol ADP phosphorylated /mg/min)	543±52	393±47*	545±31

*Each value is a mean ± S.E. of 4 to 6 experiments. * =P < 0.05 (Diabetic vs. Control). The results described here are taken from our study reported previously [59]. Diabetes in rats was induced by 65 mg/kg streptozotocin (i.v.). Insulin (2 U/day; subcutaneously; daily) was injected for 2 to 4 weeks.*

Sarcolemmal changes

Sarcolemmal channels and receptors
It is now well established that cardiac contraction is initiated when an action potential depolarizes the cell. Sarcolemma plays an important role in the generation and maintenance of transmembrane gradients of Na^+, K^+ and Ca^{2+}, which are essential for cardiac cell excitability. Operating together, sarcolemmal membrane-bound cation channels, exchange systems and cation pumps contribute to the regulation of membrane potential and the cardiac excitation-contraction coupling process [74]. Rapid calcium influx is achieved

through opening of the voltage-sensitive Ca^{2+}-channels in the plasma membrane whereas triggering the calcium-induced calcium-release depends critically on calcium stores in the SR. In cardiac cells, two types of Ca^{2+}-channels, namely L-type and T-type have been identified [75,76]. The L-type channel is the major pathway for voltage gated calcium entry into mammalian cardiac cells leading to excitation-contraction coupling and intracellular calcium transients [77,78]. Experimental findings indicate that influx of calcium via L-type channels can provide an adequate source of calcium to trigger the release of calcium from the SR. The functional status of Ca^{2+}-channels in the cell can be monitored by determining the specific binding of Ca^{2+} antagonists [75]. Nishio *et al.* [79] were the first group to report on a change in voltage-sensitive Ca^{2+}-channels of cardiac muscle crude membranes isolated from STZ-induced diabetic rats. They observed a 64% increase in the B_{max} of the calcium inhibitor [^{3}H]-PN200-110 binding sites compared to control rats without any difference in K_d; this increase in binding was found in both 6 week and 12 week STZ-diabetic rats. Two weeks after STZ treatment followed by an 8-week intensive insulin treatment normalized the increase in [^{3}H]-PN200-110 binding in streptozotocin-diabetic rats. Furthermore, unlike the membranes from diabetic heart, [^{3}H]-PN200-110 binding to control cardiac membranes was dose-dependently inhibited in the presence of verapamil.

A more recent study by Götzsche *et al.* [80] found unchanged receptor affinities in Ca^{2+}-channels in STZ-diabetic rats. However, in 4 and 7 day STZ-diabetic rats, B_{max} was depressed by about 50% compared to controls. After 6 months, B_{max} was actually increased compared to controls. Insulin treatment restored Ca^{2+}-channel B_{max} in diabetic animals. In contrast to these two studies, 3 weeks after inducing diabetes Lee *et al.* [81] reported a decrease in both ^{3}H-nitrendipine receptor number and K_d value in crude heart membrane preparations. Administration of insulin to diabetic rats for 3 weeks normalized changes in both K_d and B_{max} values. It is postulated that differences in results from various laboratories [79-81] appear to be due to the stage and intensity of diabetes and it is possible that changes in dihydropyridine binding sites are biphasic in nature. This view is supported by the fact that an increase in the density of ^{3}H-nitrendipine binding sites in heart membranes was seen in younger genetically cardiomyopathic hamsters [82,83], whereas no change was observed in older animals [84]. Differences in the results were also explained by the differences in experimental conditions employed for the preparation of membranes, but not necessarily due to differences in the ligands employed for monitoring Ca^{2+}-channels.

The decrease in density of ^{3}H-nitrendipine binding with diabetic myocardial membranes has been suggestive of a decrease in the number of voltage sensitive Ca^{2+} channels of the L-type in sarcolemma. A decrease in Ca^{2+}-influx involving Ca^{2+} channels would then serve to amplify the adverse effects of impaired SR pump [27,30] and reduced myofibrillar ATPase activities [4,5,15] on contractile force development in diabetic cardiomyopathy. Lee *et al.* [81] also observed that absolute values for contractile force development in the isolated heart preparations at different concentrations of calcium were less than those for the control preparations. It was noted, however, that the percent increase in contractile force upon increasing the perfusate calcium was higher in diabetic hearts. In fact, increased sensitivity of diabetic heart to calcium with respect to contractile force development has also been reported by other investigators [85]. This change could likely be due to an increased affinity of Ca^{2+}-channels in the diabetic sarcolemma [81]. This view would be consistent with the observation that verapamil exerted more depression of contractile force in the diabetic heart in comparison to the control. Report of increased affinity of Ca^{2+}-channels could also provide evidence to explain the occurrence of intracellular calcium overload and subsequent myocardial cell damage in the diabetic heart [26]. Overall, dramatic alterations in myocardial metabolism as a result of insulin deficiency and elevated levels of plasma glucose in diabetic animals can thus be seen to account for the observed changes in sarcolemmal Ca^{2+}-channels. Such changes may also occur due to long chain acyl derivatives which accumulate in the diabetic heart and are known to exert dramatic actions on characteristics of the cell membrane [28,86-88].

In addition to the changes in Ca^{2+}-channels, there is much evidence for alterations in cardiac receptor function and/or numbers following STZ/alloxan induced diabetes. Some of the results from our laboratory on this aspect are shown in Table 6.4. Savarese and

Berkowitz [89] were the first to report a decrease (28%) in the number of cardiac ß-adrenoceptors 8 weeks after inducing diabetes by STZ with no change in ß-adrenoceptor affinity. It was suggested that this reduction in receptor number might have contributed to the bradycardia seen in the diabetic animals [89]. Since that time, there have been several reports of diminished cardiac ß-adrenoceptor numbers, with no change in affinity, in cardiac tissue taken from rats 2 to 10 weeks after the injection of STZ [90-96] or alloxan [97]. It is likely that these changes develop gradually, because Götzsche [99] found no change in cardiac ß-adrenoceptor numbers 8 days after STZ treatment, and Latifpour

Table 6.4: Cardiac Ca^{2+}-channels and adrenergic receptors in control, diabetic and insulin-treated diabetic rats.

	Control	Diabetic	Insulin-treated diabetic
Number of Ca^{2+} channels (fmol/mg)	166±12	83±9*	146±11
Number of ß-adrenergic receptors (fmol/mg)	39±2.8	27±1.2*	38±2.6
Number of α-adrenergic receptors (fmol/mg)	55.6±1.4	34.7±2.9*	52.8±2.7

Each value is a mean ± S.E. of 3 to 6 experiments. * = P < 0.05 (Diabetic vs. Control). The results described here are taken from our studies reported previously [81,90]. Ca^{2+}-channels were measured as specific binding for ^3H-nitrendipine whereas ß- and α-adrenergic receptors were measured as specific binding for ^3H-dihydroalprenolol and 3H-dihydroergocryptin, respectively.

and McNeill [98] found a small, nonsignificant decrease in ß-adrenoceptor numbers 3 months after STZ treatment but a significant decrease after 6 months. Since Götzsche et al. [80] most recently reported down-regulation of ß-receptors as early as 4 days after STZ administration, there appears to be no consistency with regard to the time of onset of changes in ß-adrenoceptor numbers in different studies. Neither is there a clear relationship between these changes and the time of onset of bradycardia, which may occur within 4 days of STZ treatment [100]. Nonetheless, alterations in ß-adrenoceptor numbers may be relatively restricted to cardiac tissue because no change occurred in the ß-adrenoceptor populations of lung membranes from rats treated with streptozotocin [98]. In a study using refinement of earlier approaches, Kashiwagi *et al.* [101] measured concentrations of cell surface and total cell ß-adrenoceptors of cardiac myocytes 10 weeks after STZ-treatment. Although there was a 41% reduction in cell surface-binding sites, there was no difference between STZ-diabetic and control rats in total cell receptor concentrations suggesting abnormalities in ß-adrenoceptor recycling.

Chemically-induced diabetes by either alloxan or STZ may lead to uncoupling of the ß-adrenoceptor from second messenger systems. Götzsche [99] found that, in cardiac tissue taken 8 days after treatment with STZ, ß-adrenoceptor number was unaltered, but cyclic adenosine monophosphate (cAMP) accumulation in response to the ß-adrenoceptor agonist, isoprenaline, was diminished. In contrast, Atkins *et al.* [93] found that cAMP accumulation in response to isoprenaline was normal in cardiac tissue taken from rats treated 2 weeks previously with STZ, but was impaired at 4 weeks. In this study, there was a similar reduction in ß-adrenoceptor number at both times. Because no change in basal cAMP production [93,95,99] was found following STZ treatment, it was suggested that the coupling of ß-adrenoceptors to adenylyl cyclase may be abnormal. This might have been due to changes in the regulatory guanosine triphosphate binding proteins [95], because there was evidence for an increase in G_i proteins (i.e. those which inhibit adenylyl cyclase) in cardiac tissue from STZ-treated rats. Isolated papillary muscle, isolated perfused hearts, ventricular tissue and atria from STZ-treated rats as well as alloxan-treated rats also showed attenuated contractile responses to isoproterenol and noradrenaline [90,102-106]. In contrast to these studies, Austin and Chess-Williams [107] found enhanced responsiveness of isolated papillary muscles and atria from STZ-treated rats to isoprenaline and forskolin and an increase in ß-adrenoceptor number. The major difference in methodology was that Austin and Chess-Williams [107] used female rats in their study while male rats were used in all other studies with the exceptions of those by Götzsche [99] and Goyal *et al.* [105].

Because sex differences are known to occur in various cardiovascular responses mediated by the noradrenergic system [108], it is possible that STZ-treatment has different effects in male and female rats.

There are several reasons why cardiac adrenoceptor function may be altered following STZ treatment. It is possible that enhanced turnover of catecholamines in the myocardium could contribute to adrenoceptor down-regulation. Gangly *et al.* [109,110] made detailed studies of noradrenaline metabolism in cardiac tissue from STZ-treated rats. It was found that not only was cardiac noradrenaline content increased following diabetes but also noradrenaline turnover, synthesis and release were increased. The difference in noradrenaline turnover between control and STZ-diabetic rats was abolished following treatment with the ganglion blocker, pentolinium, indicating that the increase in noradrenaline turnover in diabetic rats may have been due to enhanced sympathetic nerve activity. The results of Gangly *et al.* [109] are in agreement with those of Lucas and Qirbi [111] who also found enhanced noradrenaline turnover in the ventricle of STZ-diabetic rats but are in contrast with those of Yoshida *et al.* [112,113] who obtained evidence for reduced noradrenaline turnover in hearts of STZ-diabetic rats. Thus, there remains a controversy about the effects of STZ or alloxan-induced diabetes on noradrenaline turnover.

When cardiac noradrenaline content and ß-adrenoceptor numbers were measured in the same study [93], no change in the former was found at a time when the latter was reduced. Hypothyroidism following STZ/alloxan treatment has been suggested to contribute to the diminished number of cardiac ß-adrenoceptors [92,102]. For example rats that had been thyroidectomized prior to STZ-induced diabetes developed no further reduction in ß-adrenoceptor numbers after STZ treatment [92], and administration of thyroxine (T_4) to intact rats following STZ treatment prevented the decrease in cardiac ß-adrenoceptor numbers [92]. Karasu *et al.* [102] using thyroidectomized alloxan-induced diabetic rats reported that insulin administration to these animals did not reverse the diabetes-induced changes in spontaneously beating rat atria and suggested that the thyroid hormones are needed for insulin to normalize alterations in the diabetic heart tissue. The role of hypothyroidism is, however, contentious because reductions in plasma thyroid hormone levels are not temporally related to changes in cardiac ß-adrenoceptors, and an insulin regimen that reversed the effects of STZ/alloxan on cardiac ß-adrenoceptors had no effect on plasma thyroid hormone levels [95]. Furthermore, Goyal et al. [105] found that treatment with 3,5,3'-triiodothyronine (T$_3$), at a dose that prevented the development of bradycardia, did not prevent the impairment in atrial chronotropic or inotropic responses to isoprenaline following STZ treatment. Although there is some consistency among studies in showing reductions in ß-adrenoceptor numbers and impaired coupling to second messenger systems and contractile responses, the time course of these changes and the relationship between them are not clear. In order to investigate intracellular calcium in response to ß-adrenergic stimulation, Yu et al. [114] used isolated myocytes to clarify the mechanisms involved in diabetes-induced ß-adrenergic signal transduction. The results of their studies suggested that in addition to alterations in ß-adrenoceptor function, there were post receptor defects in diabetic myocardium that could likely impair intracellular calcium in diabetic myocardium.

A reduction in cardiac α-adrenoceptor number with no changes in affinity occurs following induction of the diabetes [90, 91, 94, 98, 115]. The responsiveness of STZ-diabetic rats to α-adrenoceptor agents may also depend on the tissue used because, although contractility of isolated papillary muscle to the α$_1$-adrenoceptor agonist, methoxamine, was attenuated following STZ diabetes [90], the α$_1$-adrenoceptor-mediated chronotropic and inotropic responses of atria or ventricles isolated from STZ-diabetic rats were enhanced [104,105,116-118]. Discrepancies between the effects of STZ treatment on α-adrenoceptor numbers and responsiveness to α-adrenoceptor agonists may arise because of changes in the second messenger system. It was found that atrial calcium turnover in response to α-adrenoceptor stimulation was enhanced [117], and there were increased atrial and ventricular contractile responses to calcium [104] following the induction of diabetes. Furthermore, inositol (1,4,5)-triphosphate production in response to noradrenaline was enhanced in ventricular tissue isolated from STZ-diabetic rats [118]. In a study by Jackson et al. [117], phenylephrine in the presence or absence of the ß-adrenoceptor antagonist, timolol, was used to assess chronotropic responses. These authors observed that the response to phenylephrine alone was inhibited by timolol to a lesser extent in tissue from STZ-diabetic rats than in control animals. It was suggested that, whereas α-adrenoceptor stimulation is normally of little importance in the control of heart rate it may become increasingly important due to a diminished contribution from ß-adrenoceptor stimulation following STZ-treatment. Changes in myocardial eicosanoid production has been suggested to underline altered α-adrenoceptor function in STZ-treated rats [119]. Other factors responsible for the abnormalities in cardiac α-adrenoceptor mechanisms appear to include changes in cardiac membrane fluidity, and/or nonenzymatic glycosylation of proteins that occur during hyperglycemia [119]. Impairment of cardiac α_1-adrenoceptor signalling has also been shown to be closely associated with the diabetic state, and may be linked, at least in part, with abnormal activation of cardiac protein kinase C [115].

Muscarinic cholinergic receptors in the ventricular tissue of the heart have been found to be altered during long-term diabetes [120]; this effect was found to be dependent upon the duration of diabetes [91,98]. As was the case with ß-adrenergic receptors, muscarinic receptor density was depressed in hearts from diabetic animals but affinity was unaffected [98]. A similar observation has been reported for atrial tissue from diabetic rats; however, the decrease in muscarinic receptor density was found at earlier times after the induction of the diabetic state [120]. These changes in receptor density may partially explain alterations in the sensitivity of diabetic rat hearts to cholinergic stimulation [121]. Whether these changes in cardiac channels and receptors during the development of diabetic cardiomyopathy are due to altered gene expression is not clear at present.

Sarcolemmal pumps and transporters

The Na^+-K^+-pump, measured biochemically as Na^+-K^+-ATPase activity, is localized in the cardiac sarcolemma and is known to produce an uphill transport of sodium and potassium at the expense of ATP hydrolysis [122-124]. Regulation of intracellular sodium and potassium is vital for normal cardiac cell function as homeostasis of both these cations is necessary to maintain electrical properties of the myocardium. The concept that a rise in intracellular sodium concentration via inhibition of the Na^+-K^+-pump contributes to sarcolemmal calcium influx by activating the sarcolemmal Na^+-Ca^{2+} exchange system was emphasized by Schwartz *et al.* [123]. Thus, any change in the operation of sarcolemmal Na^+-K^+-ATPase conceivably could alter calcium movements in the cell and thus may be seen to modify cardiac contractile function. Several studies have presented evidence to suggest significant dysfunction in the diabetic cardiac plasma membrane at the site of Na^+-K^+-ATPase. Onji and Liu [125] were first to demonstrate that diabetes could be associated with a defect in the Na^+-K^+-ATPase enzyme system; this study showed that K^+-stimulated para-nitrophenyl phosphatase (K^+-pNPPase) activity in diabetic myocytes was significantly depressed in comparison to control values. Since K^+-pNPPase activity is thought to represent the dephosphorylation step of the Na^+-K^+-ATPase enzyme, this would suggest that a defect in Na^+-pumping across the sarcolemma may exist in diabetic animals. Pierce and Dhalla [126] were first to isolate a purified preparation of cardiac sarcolemma from diabetic animals in order to more closely examine the integrity of enzymes located in the plasma membrane; both ouabain-sensitive K^+-pNPPase and Na^+-K^+-ATPase activities were significantly depressed in diabetic preparations in comparison to controls. The depression in Na^+-K^+-ATPase activity correlated well with and may explain the depression of the Na^+-pump activity observed in ventricular slices from diabetic rats [127]; this change was reversible by insulin. Subsequent studies have confirmed depressions in Na^+-K^+-ATPase in experimental diabetes [128-131]. Kjeldsen *et al.* [132] reported that a depression in the number of ouabain cardiac binding sites was present with a concomitant decrease in Na^+-K^+ pump concentration in STZ-diabetic myocardium. Depressed ouabain binding in cardiac tissue during diabetes and attenuated inotropic response to ouabain have also been observed [133].

Efforts have been made by many investigators to elucidate the physiological and pathophysiological role of the sarcolemmal Na^+-Ca^{2+} exchange system in the heart since the discovery of Na^+-dependent Ca^{2+} transport [134,135]. The kinetic parameters suggest that the sarcolemmal Na^+-Ca^{2+} exchange system is capable of rapid movements of calcium in and out of the myocardial cell. In electrophysiological studies, SR calcium release was demonstrated to occur in response to graded sarcolemmal calcium influx [136] whereas the Na^+-Ca^{2+} exchange mechanism has been suggested to cause transsarcolemmal Ca^{2+}-influx subsequent to a rapid influx of sodium through the fast Na^+-channels [137]. On the other hand, Bridge et al. [138] have provided evidence to suggest that calcium

Table 6.5: Cardiac sarcolemmal alterations in control, diabetic and insulin-treated diabetic rats

	Control	Diabetic	Insulin-treated diabetic
ATP-dependent Ca^{2+} uptake (nmol Ca^{2+} /mg/min)	22.5±2.1	9.8±1.2*	16.8±2.2
Ca^{2+}-stimulated ATPase (µmol Pi/mg/hr)	13.2±0.96	5.9±0.5*	12.4±1.0
Na^+-dependent Ca^{2+} uptake (nmol Ca^{2+}/mg/ min)	42±2.6	19.8±3.8*	37±2.4
Na^+-K^+ ATPase (µmol Pi/mg/hr)	25.8±1.9	15.8±2.1*	22.0±3.1

*Each value is a mean ± S.E. of 5 to 6 experiments. * = $P < 0.05$ (Diabetic vs. Control). The results described here are taken from our study reported previously [129]. The induction of diabetes and insulin-treatments are same as given in the legend for Table 6.3.*

entering the cardiac cell during excitation is extruded by the Na^+-Ca^{2+} exchanger system. Thus sarcolemmal Na^+-Ca^{2+} exchange may be important in mediating both influx and efflux of calcium, and thereby is implicated in contractile function of the heart. The Ca^{2+}-stimulated ATPase localized in the cardiac sarcolemma and described biochemically as Ca^{2+}-stimulated, Mg^{2+}-dependent ATPase is generally believed to be involved in transsarcolemmal Ca^{2+} extrusion [45,139]. The sarcolemmal Ca^{2+}-pump is under the control of phosphorylation/ dephosphorylation reactions, mediated by Ca^{2+}-calmodulin-dependent and cAMP-dependent protein kinases [140,141]. This mechanism of regulation may be important in balancing the increased influx of calcium due to ß-adrenoceptor activation of the slow Ca^{2+}-channels. Sarcolemmal Na^{+}-Ca^{2+} exchange and Ca^{2+}-pump activities (measured biochemically as Ca^{2+}-stimulated ATPase and ATP-dependent Ca^{2+} uptake) have been shown to be depressed in chronic diabetes and normalized by insulin administration [128-130,142]. Changes in heart sarcolemmal Ca^{2+}-transport and ATPase activities in diabetic heart and their reversibility by insulin (Table 6.5) provide further that the sarcolemmal membrane is remodelled during the development of diabetic cardiomyopathy [137]. However, no information regarding changes in gene expression with respect to sarcolemmal Na^{+}-Ca^{2+} exchanger, Na^{+}-K^{+}-ATPase or Ca^{2+}-pump in diabetic heart is available in the literature.

One of the mechanisms for the movement of sodium into the myocardium is through sodium-hydrogen exchange [143]. This cation transport system has been identified in myocardial cells and in isolated, cardiac sarcolemmal membrane vesicles [143,144]. The transporter is electroneutral and sensitive to various cations [144]. In addition to its role in controlling sodium entry into the myocardial cell, the accompanying hydrogen efflux may also play a role in the steady-state maintenance of intracellular pH (pH_i). A study by Lagadic-Gossmann et al. [145] observed no difference between the steady-state pH_i values recorded from diabetic or normal papillary muscle. On the other hand, the amplitude of the acidification induced by withdrawal of NH_4^{+} was markedly increased in diabetic papillary muscles vs. control; there was a marked slowing down of the recovery from acidosis in diabetics. These early findings suggested that diabetes is associated with a change in the activity of the amiloride-sensitive Na^{+}-H^{+} exchange. In isolated sarcolemmal vesicles from STZ-diabetic rats, Pierce et al. [130] noted a striking depression (67%) in cardiac sarcolemmal Na^{+}-H^{+} exchange compared to control. These results represented the first observation of an alteration in Na^{+}-H^{+} exchange in cardiac sarcolemma during a diseased state. These results suggest that both pH_i and intracellular sodium may also be disturbed in the myocardium during diabetes. Altered Na^{+}-H^{+} exchange activities in diabetic rat hearts can have a profound effect on pH_i and functional recovery in the early stages of reperfusion from ischemic challenge [146].

Cardiac membrane lipid composition

Lipids, proteins and carbohydrates are three major important components that constitute the cell membrane. These three components have received some attention as possible determinants of cardiomyopathy in diabetes mellitus. A change in the composition of the sarcolemmal membrane, or other membrane systems, has two important ramifications. A change in the membrane microenvironment and its biophysical properties can influence: (i) its permeability characteristics and, (ii) modulate enzymatic activities [147]. Such changes will have immediate and dramatic effects on cardiac function, viability, and integrity. Protein changes are most obvious to induce alterations in enzyme activity. However, gross qualitative and quantitative protein composition when analyzed by protein separation with SDS polyacrylamide gel electrophoresis [148] did not reveal any major changes in the sarcolemmal membrane as a function of the diabetic state, although a significant increase in protein of approximately 70,000 daltons was identified [148]. Major alterations in the lipid composition of sarcolemma isolated from hearts of diabetic rats have been demonstrated [126,129,148]. Phosphatidylethanolamine and diphosphatidylglycerol concentrations were depressed whereas lysophosphatidylcholine levels were increased significantly in diabetic preparations in comparison to control values; other phospholipids were unaltered. These changes in phospholipid composition of the cardiac sarcolemma are thought to be important to cellular function and integrity during diabetes. Lysophosphatidylcholine accumulation in the heart has been associated with electrophysiological abnormalities [149] and permeability changes [150]. Therefore, the increase in lysophosphatidylcholine concentration in diabetic sarcolemma may perhaps adequately explain the alterations in electrical activity and an increase in sarcolemmal membrane leakiness in diabetic hearts [151-153].

Phosphatidylethanolamine degradation has also been shown to be associated with defects in sarcolemmal permeability in the myocardium [154]. It is thus possible, that the increase in lyso-phosphatidylethanolamine and the decrease in phosphatidyl-ethanolamine could be important factors in altering the sarcolemmal membrane permeability in the heart from diabetic animals. In addition, an increased level of lysophosphatidylcholine has been shown to inhibit Na^+-K^+-ATPase activity [155], and therefore, could be causally related to the depression in Na^+-K^+-ATPase [126] and Na^+-pump activities [127] in diabetic cardiomyopathy. Lysophosphatidylcholine has also been shown to inhibit Na^+-Ca^{2+} exchange activity; this suggests that the accumulation of lipid metabolites may produce heart dysfunction by modifying calcium movements across the sarcolemmal membrane [156]. The change in diphosphatidylglycerol content may have further relevance to the decrease in sarcolemmal calcium binding in the diabetic preparations [148]. A recent study has examined the molecular species composition of heart sarcolemmal phosphatidylcholine in diabetic cardiomyopathy [157]. These investigators reported that phosphatidylcholine from STZ-diabetic rat heart sarcolemma was highly enriched with 18:0/22:6 and 16:0/22:16 species; insulin normalized these values. Minor changes in arachidonic acid-containing phosphatidylcholine were also observed. It was suggested that the observed changes in the molecular species composition of diabetic sarcolemmal phosphatidylcholine, sarcolemma content may lead to abnormal diacylglycerol species. Their observations further indicated that there may well be alterations in the PKC-dependent phosphorylation processes in the diabetic heart.

The phospholipid N-methylation has been suggested to be important in changing several membrane-associated functions [158] including the control of calcium fluxes in the myocardium [159-161]. Phosphatidylethanolamine N-methylation has been shown to increase Ca^{2+}-pump activities in heart sarcolemma and SR [160,161]. Studies with 6-week STZ-diabetic rats have shown that phosphatidylethanolamine N-methylation was defective in cardiac sarcolemmal membranes [162,163] and altered in other subcellular organelles, such as the mitochondria and sarcoplasmic reticulum [163]; these alterations were reversed with insulin treatment. Cholesterol composition of the sarcolemma isolated from hearts of diabetic rats was also found to be altered [126,129,148]. In these studies, total cholesterol content has been shown to increase in diabetic preparations; this is likely to be due to the elevation in plasma cholesterol concentration in these diabetic animals. Since alterations in membrane cholesterol content are known to have dramatic effects on enzyme activities [147], elevated cholesterol levels in sarcolemma from diabetic animals may induce changes in the sarcolemmal enzyme activities.

Carbohydrate residues associated with the basement membrane component of the cardiac sarcolemmal membrane from diabetic rats were also found to be altered. Specifically, the sialic acid residues in the sarcolemma were significantly reduced during diabetes [148]; this change in membrane composition could be normalized if diabetic animals were made euglycemic with chronic insulin administration. Removal of sialic acid residues from the sarcolemmal membrane has been closely associated with an increase in membrane permeability [164,165]. Thus, it is possible, that a decrease in sialic acid content in cardiac sarcolemma from diabetic rats may alter permeability characteristics; this would correlate well with the *in vivo* evidence of change in integrity of hearts from diabetic animals [57]. A "leaky" plasma membrane may also explain reports of altered cation contents [166] in myocardium from diabetic animals. The depression in sarcolemmal sialic acid content can relate to an observed decrease in passive calcium binding to this membrane during diabetes [148]. It should be noted that sialic acid residues represent a source of fixed net negative charge on the external surface of the sarcolemma. Because of this, they are capable of attracting positively charged calcium ions; the depression in sialic acid content, therefore, may be associated with the decrease in Ca^{2+}-binding to the sarcolemma. It is, however, important to point out that conflicting data exist regarding the importance of sialic acid residues in sarcolemmal Ca^{2+}-binding [167] and it appears that the alteration in glycoprotein residues may not be the only factor responsible for the defect in membrane Ca^{2+}-binding. In this regard, it is also indicated that acidic phospholipids are capable of binding large quantities of calcium [168]. Therefore, the decrease in content of the acidic phospholipid and diphosphatidylglycerol may also be partially responsible for the depression in calcium binding to cardiac sarcolemma isolated from diabetic rats [148].

Summary

In this article we have reviewed the existing literature concerning changes in subcellular organelles such as myofibrils, SR, mitochondria and sarcolemma during the development of diabetic cardiomyopathy. It appears that the impaired ability of diabetic heart to contract and relax is mainly due to depressed myofibrillar Ca^{2+}-stimulated ATPase and SR Ca^{2+}-pump activities, respectively. The defects in myofibrils seem to be associated with changes in sulfhydryl-group reactivity and a shift in myosin isoenzymes as a consequence of changes in gene expression. On the other hand, impairment in the SR Ca^{2+}-pump activities appears to be associated with the accumulation of some lipid metabolites in the SR membrane without any changes in the gene expression. During early stages of diabetes, mitochondrial Ca^{2+}-transport seems to be normal and thus these organelles may serve to protect the myocardial cell from the occurrence of intracellular Ca^{2+}-overload. However, excessive accumulation of calcium in mitochondria appears to impair their function for generating energy through oxidative phosphorylation as well as for transporting calcium and these changes can be seen to further deteriorate the function of diabetic heart. Although dramatic changes in the sarcolemmal membrane with respect to cation transport and translocation have been identified in the diabetic heart, the functional significance of these alterations is poorly understood. Alterations in the composition of phospholipids, cholesterol and sialic acid residues may explain some of the changes in the sarcolemmal Na^+-K^+ ATPase, Na^+-Ca^{2+} exchange, Ca^{2+}-pump, Ca^{2+}-channels and adrenergic receptors in the diabetic heart; however, molecular mechanisms in this regard need to be investigated. Nonetheless, it is evident that there occurs a remodelling of subcellular organelles during the development of diabetic cardiomyopathy and it is crucial to correct these subcellular defects for the treatment of heart dysfunction in chronic diabetes.

Acknowledgments

The research reported in this paper was supported by a grant from the Canadian Diabetes Association and The Vehicle Racing Commemorative Foundation, Tokyo.

References

1. Gergely J. Some aspects of the role of the sarcoplasmic reticulum and the tropomyosin-troponin system in the control of muscle contraction by calcium ions. *Circ. Res.* **35** (Suppl III): 74-82, 1974.

2. Scheuer J and Bhan AK. Cardiac contractile proteins. Adenosine triphosphate activity and physiological function. *Circ. Res.* **45**: 1-12, 1979.

3. Barany M. ATPase activity of myosin correlated with speed of muscle shortening. *J. Gen. Physiol.* **50** (Suppl): 197-218, 1967.

4. Pierce GN and Dhalla NS. Cardiac myofibrillar ATPase activity in diabetic rats. *J. Mol. Cell. Cardiol.* **13**: 1063-1069, 1981.

5. Pierce GN and Dhalla NS. Mechanisms of the defect in cardiac myofibrillar function during diabetes. *Am. J. Physiol.* **248**: E170-E175, 1985.

6. Afzal N, Pierce GN, Elimban V, Beamish RE and Dhalla NS. Influence of verapamil on some subcellular defects in diabetic cardiomyopathy. *Am. J. Physiol.* **256**: E453-E458, 1989.

7. Pollack PS, Malhotra A, Fein FS and Scheuer J. Effects of diabetes on cardiac contractile proteins in rabbits and reversal with insulin. *Am. J. Physiol.* **20**: H448-H454, 1986.

8. Bhimji S, Godin DV and McNeill JH. Biochemical and functional changes in hearts from rabbits with diabetes. *Diabetologia* **28**: 452-457, 1985.

9. Pierce GN, Beamish RE and Dhalla NS (eds). *Heart Dysfunction in Diabetes.* Boca Raton, FL: CRC, 1988, p. 1-245.

10. Solaro RJ, Wise RM, Shiner JS and Briggs FN. Calcium requirements for cardiac myofibrillar activation. *Circ. Res.* **34**: 525-530, 1974.

11. Dillmann WH. Diabetes mellitus induces changes in cardiac myosin of the rat. *Diabetes* **29**: 579-582, 1980.

12. Schaible TF, Malhotra A, Bauman WA and Scheuer J. Left ventricular function after chronic insulin treatment in diabetic and normal rats. *J. Mol. Cell. Cardiol.* **15**: 445-458, 1983.

13. Garber DW and Neely JR. Decreased myocardial function and myosin ATPase in hearts from diabetic rats. *Am. J. Physiol.* **244**: H586-H591, 1983.

14. Garber DW, Everett AW and Neely JR. Cardiac function and myosin ATPase in diabetic rats treated with insulin, T3 and T4. *Am. J. Physiol.* **244**: H592-H598, 1983.

15. Malhotra A, Penpargkul S, Fein FS, Sonnenblick EH and Scheuer J. The effect of streptozotocin-induced diabetes in rats on cardiac contractile proteins. *Circ. Res.* **49**: 1243-1250, 1981.

16. Dillmann WH. Influence of thyroid hormone administration on myosin ATPase activity and myosin isoenzyme distribution in the heart of diabetic rats. *Metabolism* **31**: 199-204, 1982.

17. Rupp H, Elimban V and Dhalla NS. Diabetes-like action of intermittant fasting on sarcoplasmic reticulum Ca^{2+}-pump ATPase and myosin isoenzymes can be prevented by sucrose. *Biochem. Biophys. Res. Commun.* **164**: 319-325, 1989.

18. Rupp H, Jacob R and Dhalla NS. Signal transduction of myosin heavy-chain expression in the diabetic heart. In: *The Diabetic Heart,* Nagano M and Dhalla NS (eds). Raven Press, Ltd. New York 1991, p.271-279.

19. Hoh JFY, McGrath PA and Hale PT. Electrophoretic analysis of multiple forms of rat cardiac myosin: Effects of hypophysectomy and thyroxine replacement. *J. Mol. Cell. Cardiol.* **10**: 1053-1076, 1978.

20. Schwartz K, Lecarpentier Y, Martin JL, Lompre AM, Mercadier JJ and Swynghedauw B. Myosin isoenzyme

distribution correlates with speed of myocardial contraction. *J. Mol. Cell. Cardiol.* **13**: 1071-1075, 1981.

21. Boheler KR, Chassagne C, Martin X, Wisnewsky C and Schwartz K. Cardiac expressions of alpha- and ß-myosin heavy chains and sarcomeric alpha-actins are regulated through transcriptional mechanisms. *J. Biol. Chem.* **267**: 12979-12985, 1992.

22. Dillman WH. Diabetes-induced changes in specific proteins and mRNAs in the rat heart. In: *The Diabetic Heart*, Nagano M and Dhalla NS (eds), Raven Press, Ltd, New York. 1991, p. 263-270.

23. Fabiato A. Calcium release in skinned cardiac cells: Variations with species, tissues, and development. *Fed. Proc.* **41**: 2238-2244, 1982.

24. Carafoli E. Intracellular Ca^{2+} homeostasis. *Ann. Rev. Biochem.* **56**: 395-433, 1987.

25. Inesi G. Mechanism of calcium transport. *Ann. Rev. Physiol.* **47**: 573-601, 1985.

26. Dhalla NS, Pierce GN, Innes IR and Beamish RE. Pathogenesis of cardiac dysfunction in diabetes mellitus. *Can. J. Cardiol.* **1**: 263-281, 1985.

27. Penpargkul S, Fein F, Sonnenblick EH and Scheuer J. Depressed sarcoplasmic reticular function for diabetic rats. *J. Mol. Cell. Cardiol.* **13**: 303-309, 1981.

28. Lopaschuk GD, Katz S and McNeill JH. The effect of alloxan- and streptozotocin-induced diabetes on calcium transport in rat cardiac sarcoplasmic reticulum. The possible involvement of long chain acyl-carnitines. *Can. J. Physiol. Pharmacol.* **61**: 439-448, 1983.

29. Lopaschuk GD, Tahiliani AG, Vadlamudi RVSV, Katz S and McNeill JH. Cardiac sarcoplasmic reticulum function in insulin- or carnitine-treated diabetic rats. *Am. J. Physiol.* **245**: H969-H976, 1984.

30. Ganguly PK, Pierce GN, Dhalla KS and Dhalla NS. Defective sarcoplasmic reticular calcium transport in diabetic cardiomyopathy. *Am. J. Physiol.* **244**: E528-E535, 1983.

31. Pierce GN, Ganguly PK, Dzurba A and Dhalla NS. Modification of the function of cardiac subcellular organelles by insulin. *Adv. Myocardiol.* **6**: 113-125, 1985.

32. Suko J. The calcium pump of cardiac sarcoplasmic reticulum. Functional alterations at different levels of thyroid state in rabbits. *J. Physiol. (London)* **228**: 563-569, 1973.

33. Lopaschuk GD, Eibschutz B, Katz S and McNeill JH. Depression of calcium transport in sarcoplasmic reticulum from diabetic rats: Lack of involvement by specific regulatory mediators. *Gen. Pharmacol.* **15**: 1-5, 1984.

34. Feuvray D, Idell-Wenger JA and Neely JR. Effects of ischemia on rat myocardial function and metabolism in diabetes. *Circ. Res.* **44**: 322-329, 1979.

35. Pitts B, Tate CA, Van Winkle B, Wood TM and Entman ML. Palmitoylcarnitine inhibition of the calcium pump in cardiac sarcoplasmic reticulum: A possible role in myocardial ischemia. *Life Sci.* **23**: 391-402, 1978.

36. Dhalla NS, Kolar F, Shah KR and Ferrari R. Effects of some L-carnitine derivatives on heart membrane ATPases. *Cardiovasc. Drugs Therapy* **5**: 25-30, 1991.

37. Paulson DJ, Schmidt MJ, Traxler JS, Ramacci MT and Shug AL. Improvement of myocardial function in diabetic rats after treatment with L-carnitine. *Metabolism* **33**: 358-363, 1984.

38. Ferrari R, Shah KR, Hata T, Beamish RE and Dhalla NS. Subcellular defect in diabetic myocardium: Influence of propionyl L-carnitine on Ca^{2+} transport. In: Nagano M and Dhalla NS, eds. *The Diabetic Heart*. New York, Raven Press, 1991, p. 167-181.

39. Afzal N, Ganguly PK, Dhalla KS, Pierce GN, Singal PK and Dhalla NS. Beneficial effects of verapamil in diabetic cardiomyopathy. *Diabetes* **37**: 936-942, 1988.

40. Katagiri T, Umezawa Y, Suwa Y, Geshi E, Yanagishita T and Yaida M. Biochemical and morphological alterations in cardiac myocytes in streptozotocin-induced diabetic rats. In: *Cardiovascular Disease in Diabetes*, Nagano M, Mochizuki S and Dhalla NS (eds), Kluwer Academic Publishers, Norwell, MA, 1992, p. 139-153.

41. Russ M, Reinauer H and Eckel J. Diabetes-induced decrease in the mRNA coding for sarcoplasmic reticulum Ca^{2+}-ATPase in adult rat cardiomyocytes. *Biochem. Biophys. Res. Commun.* **178**: 906-912, 1991.

42. Zarain-Herzberg A, Yano K, Elimban V and Dhalla NS. Cardiac sarcoplasmic reticulum Ca^{2+}-ATPase expression in streptozotocin-induced diabetic rat heart. *Biochem. Biophys. Res. Commun.* **203**: 113-120, 1994.

43. Scarpa A and Grazziotti, P. Mechanisms for intracellular calcium regulation in the heart. I. Stopped-flow measurements of Ca^{2+} uptake by mitochondria. *J. Gen. Physiol.* **62**: 756-772, 1973.

44. Dhalla NS, Das PK and Sharma GP. Subcellular basis of cardiac contractile failure. *J. Mol. Cell. Cardiol.* **10**: 363-383, 1978.

45. Dhalla NS, Dixon IMC and Beamish RE. Biochemical basis of heart function and contractile failure. *J. Appl. Cardiol.* **6**: 7-30, 1991.

46. Tanaka Y, Konno N and Kako KJ. Mitochondrial dysfunction observed in situ in cardiomyocytes of rats in experimental diabetes. *Cardiovasc. Res.* **26**: 409-414, 1992.

47. Dhalla NS, Pierce GN, Panagia V, Singal PK and Beamish RE. Calcium movements in relation to heart function. *Basic Res. Cardiol.* **77**: 117-139, 1982.

48. Jackson CV, McGrath GM, Tahiliani AG, Vadlamudi RVSV and McNeill JH. A functional and ultra-structural analysis of experimental diabetic rat myocardium: Manifestation of a cardiomyopathy. *Diabetes* **34**: 876-883, 1985.

49. Seager MJ, Singal PK, Orchard R, Pierce GN and Dhalla NS. Cardiac cell damage: A primary myocardial disease in streptozotocin-induced chronic diabetes. *Br. J. Exp. Pathol.* **65**: 613-623, 1984.

50. Goranson ES and Erulkar SD. The effect of insulin on the aerobic phosphorylation of creatine in tissues from alloxan-diabetic rats. *Arch. Biochem.* **24**: 40-48, 1949.

51. Kerbey AL, Randle PJ, Cooper RH, Whitehouse S, Pask HT and Denton RM. Regulation of pyruvate dehydrogenase in rat heart. *Biochem. J.* **154**: 327-348, 1967.

52. Puckett SW and Reddy WJ. A decrease in the malate-aspartate shuttle and glutamate translocase activity in heart mitochondria from alloxan-diabetic rats. *J. Mol. Cell. Cardiol.* **11**: 173-187, 1979.

53. Wieland O, Siess E, Schulze-Wethmar FH, Van Funcke HG and Winton B. Active and inactive forms of pyruvate dehydrogenase in rat heart and kidney: Effects of diabetes, fasting and refeeding on pyruvate dehydrogenase interconversion. *Arch. Biochem. Biophys.* **143**: 593-601, 1971.

54. Flutson NJ, Kerbey AL, Randle PJ and Sugden PH. Conversion of inactive (phosphorylated) pyruvate dehydrogenase complex into active complex by the phosphate reaction in heart mitochondria is inhibited by alloxan-diabetes or starvation in the rat. *Biochem. J.* **173**: 669-675, 1978.

55. Haugaard ES and Haugaard N. Diabetic Metabolism 1. Carbohydrate utilization and high energy phosphate formation in heart homogenate from normal and alloxan-diabetic rats. *J. Biol. Chem.* **239**: 705-709, 1964.

56. Chen V and Ianuzzo CD. Dosage effect of streptozotocin on rat tissue enzyme activities and glycogen concentration. *Can. J. Physiol. Pharmacol.* **60**: 1251-1256, 1982.

57. Kuo TH, Moore KH, Giacomelli F and Weiner J. Defective oxidative metabolism of heart mitochondria from genetically diabetic mice. *Diabetes* **32**: 781-787, 1983.

58. Kuo TH, Giacomelli F and Weiner J. Oxidative metabolism of Polytron versus Nagarse mitochondria in hearts of genetically diabetic mice. *Biochim. Biophys. Acta* **806**: 9-15, 1985.

59. Pierce GN and Dhalla NS. Heart mitochondrial function in chronic experimental diabetes in rats. *Can. J. Cardiol.* **1**: 48-54, 1985.

60. Opie LH, Tansey MJ and Kennelly BM. The heart in diabetes mellitus. I. Biochemical basis for myocardial dysfunction. *S. Afr. Med. J.* **56**: 207-235, 1979.

61. Pieper GM, Salhany JM, Murray WJ, Wu ST and Eliot RS. Lipid-mediated impairment of normal energy metabolism in the isolated perfused diabetic rat heart studied by phosphorus-31 NMR and chemical extraction. *Biochim. Biophys. Acta* **83**: 229-240, 1984.

62. Pieper GM, Murray WJ, Salhany JM, Wu ST and Eliot RS. Salient effects of L-carnitine on adenine-nucleotide loss and coenzyme A acylation in the diabetic heart perfused with excess palmitic acid. A phosphorus-31 NMR and chemical extract study. *Biochim. Biophys. Acta.* **803**: 241-252, 1984.

63. Pieper GM, Salhany JM, Murray WJ, Wu ST and Eliot RS. Abnormal phosphocreatine metabolism in perfused diabetic hearts. *Biochem. J.* **210**: 477-481, 1983.

64. Allison TB, Bruttig SP, Crass MF, Eliot RS and Shipp JC. Reduced high-energy phosphate levels in rat hearts. I. Effects of alloxan diabetes. *Am. J. Physiol.* **230**: 1744-1750, 1976.

65. Miller TB. Cardiac performance of isolated perfused hearts from alloxan diabetic rats. *Am. J. Physiol.* **236**: H808-H812, 1979.

66. Tan BH, Wilson GL and Schaffer SW. Effect of tolbutamide on myocardial metabolism and mechanical performance of the diabetic rat. *Diabetes* **33**: 1138-1145, 1984.

67. Veksler VI, Murat I and Ventura-Clapier R. Creatine kinase and mechanical and mitochondrial functions in hereditary and diabetic cardiomyopathies. *Can. J. Physiol. Pharmacol.* **69**: 852-858, 1991.

68. Savabi F and Kirsch A. Alterations in the phosphocreatine energy shuttle components in diabetic rat heart. *J. Mol. Cell. Cardiol.* **23**: 1323-1333, 1991.

69. Saks VA, Rosenhtraukh LV, Smirnov VN and Chazov EI. Role of creatine phosphokinase in cellular function and metabolism. *Can. J. Physiol. Pharmacol.* **56**: 691-706, 1978.

70. Popovich BK, Boheler KR and Dillmann WH. Diabetes decreases creatine kinase enzyme activity and mRNA level in the rat heart. *Am. J. Physiol.* **257**: E573-E577, 1989.

71. Tanaka Y, Konno N and Kako KJ. Mitochondrial dysfunction observed in situ in cardiomyocytes of rats in experimental diabetes. *Cardiovasc. Res.* **26**: 409-414, 1992.

72. Murphy JG, Smith TW and Marsh JD. Calcium flux measurements during hypoxia in cultured heart cells. *J. Mol. Cell. Cardiol.* **19**: 271-279, 1987.

73. Langer GA, Frank JS, Rich TL and Orner FB. Calcium exchange, structure and function in cultured adult myocardial cells. *Am. J. Physiol.* **252**: H314-H324, 1987.

74. Fabiato A. Time and calcium dependence of activation and inactivation of calcium-induced release of calcium from the sarcoplasmic reticulum of a skinned canine cardiac Purkinje cell. *J. Gen. Physiol.* **85**: 247-289, 1985.

75. Nilius B, Hess P, Lansman JB and Tsien RW. A novel type of cardiac calcium channel in ventricular cells. *Nature* **316**: 443-446, 1985.

76. Bean BP. Classes of calcium channels in vertebrate cells. *Ann. Rev. Physiol.* **51**: 367-384, 1989.

77. Cleemann L and Morad M. Role of Ca^{2+} channel in cardiac excitation contraction in the rat: Evidence from Ca^{2+} transients and contraction. *J. Physiol. (Lond.)* **432**: 283-312, 1991.

78. Callewaert G. Excitation-contraction coupling in mammalian cardiac cells. *Cardiovasc. Res.* **26**: 923-932, 1992.

79. Nishio Y, Kahiwagi A, Ogawa T, Asahina T, Ikebuchi M, Kodama M and Shigeta Y. Increase in [^{3}H] PN200-110 binding to cardiac muscle membrane in streptozotocin-induced diabetic rats. *Diabetes* **39**: 1064-1069, 1990.

80. Götzsche LB-H, Flyvbjerg A, Gronbaek H and Götzsche O. Quantitative changes in myocardial Ca^{2+}-channels and ß-receptors in long- vs. short-term streptozotocin diabetic rats. *J. Mol. Cell. Cardiol.* **26**: LXXIV, 1994.

81. Lee SL, Ostadalova I, Kolar F and Dhalla NS. Alterations in Ca^{2+}-channels during the development of diabetic cardiomyopathy. *Mol. Cell. Biochem.* **109**: 173-179, 1992.

82. Wagner JA, Reynolds IJ, Weisman HF, Dudeck P, Weisfeldt ML and Snyder SH. Calcium antagonist receptors in cardiomyopathic hamsters. Selective increases in heart, muscle, brain. *Science* **232**: 515-518, 1987.

83. Finkel MS, Marks ES, Patterson RE, Speir EH, Stadman KA and Keiser HR. Correlation of changes in cardiac calcium channels with hemodynamics in Syrian hamster cardiomyopathy and heart failure. *Life Sci.* **41**: 153-159, 1987.

84. Wagner JA, Weisman HF, Snowman AM, Reynold IJ, Weisfeldt ML and Snyder SH. Alterations in calcium antagonist receptor and sodium-calcium exchange in cardiomyopathic hamster tissues. *Circ. Res.* **65**: 205-214, 1989.

85. Bielefeld DR, Pace CS and Boshell BR. Altered sensitivity of chronic diabetic rat heart to calcium. *Am. J. Physiol.* **245**: E560-E567, 1983.

86. Adams RJ, Cohen DW, Gupta J, Johnson D, Wallick ET, Tang T and Schwartz AS. In vitro effects of palmitoylcarnitine on cardiac plasma membrane Na-K-ATPase and sarcoplasmic reticulum Ca^{2+} ATPase and Ca^{2+} transport. *J. Biol. Chem.* **254**: 12404-12410, 1979.

87. Wood JM, Bush B, Pitts BJR and Schwartz A. Inhibition of bovine heart Na^+, K^+-ATPase by palmitylcarnitine and palmityl CoA. *Biochem. Biophys. Res. Commun.* **74**: 677-684, 1977.

88. Kramer JH and Weglicki WB. Inhibition of sarcolemmal Na-K-ATPase by palmitoylcarnitine: Potentiation by propranolol. *Am. J. Physiol.* **284**: H75-H81, 1985.

89. Savarese JJ and Berkowitz BA. ß-Adrenergic receptor decrease in diabetic rat hearts. *Life Sci.* **25**: 2075-2078, 1979.

90. Heyliger CE, Pierce GN, Singal PK, Beamish RE and Dhalla NS. Cardiac alpha- and beta-adrenergic receptor alterations in

diabetic cardiomyopathy. *Basic Res. Cardiol.* **77**: 610-618, 1982.

91. Williams RS, Schaible TF, Scheuer J and Kennedy R. Effects of experimental diabetes on adrenergic and cholinergic receptors of rat myocardium. *Diabetes* **32**: 881-886, 1983.

92. Sundaresan PR, Sharma VK, Gingold SI and Banerjee SP. Decreased ß-adrenergic receptors in rat heart in streptozotocin-induced diabetes: Role of thyroid hormones. *Endocrinology* **114**: 1358-1363, 1984.

93. Atkins FL, Dowell RT and Love S. ß-adrenergic receptors, adenylate cyclase activity, and cardiac dysfunction in the diabetic rat. *J. Cardiovasc. Pharmacol.* **7**: 66-70, 1985.

94. Bitar MS, Koulu M, Rapoport SI and Linnoila M. Adrenal catecholamine metabolism and myocardial adrenergic receptors in streptozotocin diabetic rats. *Biochem. Pharmacol.* **36**: 1011-1016, 1987.

95. Nishio Y, Kashiwagi A, Kida Y, Kodama M, Abe N, Saeki Y and Shigeta Y. Deficiency of cardiac ß-adrenergic receptor in streptozotocin-induced diabetic rats. *Diabetes* **37**: 1181-1187, 1988.

96. Ramanadham S and Tenner TE, Jr. Alterations in the myocardial ß-adrenoceptor system of streptozotocin-diabetic rats. *Eur. J. Pharmacol.* **136**: 337-389, 1987.

97. Ingebretsen CG, Hawelu-Johnson C and Ingebretsen WR, Jr. Alloxan-induced diabetes reduces ß-adrenergic receptor number without affecting adenylate cyclase in rat ventricular membranes. *J. Cardiovasc. Pharmacol.* **5**: 454-461, 1983.

98. Latifpour J and McNeill JH. Cardiac autonomic receptors: Effects of long-term experimental diabetes. *J. Pharmacol. Exp. Ther.* **230**: 242-249, 1984.

99. Götzsche O. The adrenergic beta-receptor adenylate cyclase system in heart and lymphocytes from streptozotocin-diabetic rats. *Diabetes* **32**: 1110-1116, 1983.

100. Tomlinson KC, Gardiner SM and Bennett T. Diabetes mellitus in Brattleboro rats: Cardiovascular, fluid, and electrolyte status. *Am. J. Physiol.* **256**: R1279-R1285, 1989.

101. Kashiwagi A, Nishio Y, Saeki Y, Kida Y, Kodama M and Shigeta Y. Plasma membrane-specific deficiency in cardiac ß-adrenergic receptor in streptozotocin-diabetic rats. *Am. J. Physiol.* **257**: E127-E132, 1989.

102. Karasu C, Ozturk Y, Altan N, Yildizoglu-Ari N, Ikizler C and Altan YM. Thyroid hormones mediated effect of insulin on alloxan diabetic rat atria. *Gen. Pharmacol.* **21**: 735-740, 1990.

103. Ingebretsen WR, Peralta C, Monsher M, Wagner LK and Ingebretsen CG. Diabetes alters the myocardial cAMP protein kinase cascade system. *Am. J. Physiol.* **240**: H375-382, 1981.

104. Yu Z and McNeill JH. Altered inotropic responses in diabetic cardiomyopathy and hypertensive-diabetic cardiomyopathy. *J. Pharmacol. Exp. Ther.* **257**: 64-71, 1991.

105. Goyal RK, Rodrigues B and McNeill JH. Effect of tri-iodothyronine on cardiac responses to adrenergic-agonists in STZ-induced diabetic rats. *Gen. Pharmacol.* **18**: 357-362, 1987.

106. Sato N, Hashimoto H, Takiguchi Y and Nakashima M. Altered responsiveness to sympathetic nerve stimulation and agonist of isolated left atria of diabetic rats: No evidence for involvement of hypothyroidism. *J. Pharmacol. Exp. Ther.* **248**: 367-371, 1989.

107. Austin CE and Chess-Williams R. Diabetes-induced changes in cardiac ß-adrenoceptor responsiveness: Effects of aldose reductase inhibition with ponalrestat. *Br. J. Pharmacol.* **102**: 478-482, 1991.

108. Freedman RR, Sabharwal SC and Desai N. Sex differences in peripheral vascular adrenergic receptors. *Circ. Res.* **61**: 581-585, 1987.

109. Ganguly PK, Beamish RE, Dhalla KS, Innes IR and Dhalla NS. Norepinephrine storage, distribution, and release in diabetic cardiomyopathy. *Am. J. Physiol.* **252**: E734-E739, 1987.

110. Ganguly PK, Dhalla KS, Innes IR, Beamish RE and Dhalla NS. Altered norepinephrine turnover and metabolism in diabetic cardiomyopathy. *Circ. Res.* **59**: 684-693, 1986.

111. Lucas PD and Qirbi A. Tissue noradrenaline and the polyol pathway in experimentally diabetic rats. *Br. J. Pharmacol.* **97**: 347-352, 1989.

112. Yoshida T, Nishioka H, Nakamura Y and Kondo M. Reduced noradrenaline turnover in streptozotocin-induced diabetic rats. *Diabetologia* **28**: 692-696, 1985.

113. Yoshida T, Nishioka H, Yoshioka K, Nakano K, Kondo M and Terashima H. Effect of aldose reductase inhibitor ONO 2235 on reduced sympathetic nervous system activity and peripheral nerve disorders in STZ-induced diabetic rats. *Diabetes* **36**: 6-13, 1987.

114. Yu Z, Quamme GA and McNeill JH. Depressed $[Ca^{2+}]i$ responses to isoproterenol and cAMP in isolated cardiomyocytes from experimental diabetic rats. *Am. J. Physiol.* **266**: H2334-H2342, 1994.

115. Tanaka Y, Kashiwagi A, Saeki Y and Shigeta Y. Abnormalities in cardiac alpha1-adrenoceptor and its signal transduction in streptozotocin-induced diabetic rats. *Am. J. Physiol.* **263**: E425-E429, 1992.

116. Canga L and Sterin-Borda L. Hypersensitivity to methoxamine in atria isolated from streptozotocin-induced diabetic rats. *Br. J. Pharmacol.* **87**: 156-165, 1986.

117. Jackson CV, McGrath GM and McNeill JH. Alterations in alpha1-adrenoceptor stimulation of isolated atria from experimental diabetic rats. *Can. J. Physiol. Pharmacol.* **64**: 145-151, 1986.

118. Xiang H and McNeill JH. Calcium uptake activity of cardiac sarcoplasmic reticulum in myoinositol-treated diabetic rats. *Gen. Pharmacol.* **21**: 251-254, 1990.

119. Tomlinson KC, Gardiner SM, Hebden RA and Bennett T. Functional consequences of streptozotocin-induced diabetes mellitus, with particular reference to the cardiovascular system. *Pharmacol. Rev.* **44**: 103-150, 1992.

120. Carrier GO, Edwards AD and Aronstam RS. Cholinergic supersensitivity and decreased number of muscarinic receptors in atria from short-term diabetic rats. *J. Mol. Cell. Cardiol.* **16**: 963-965, 1984.

121. Vadlamudi RVSV and McNeill JH. Effect of alloxan-streptozotocin-induced diabetes on isolated rat heart responsiveness to carbachol. *J. Pharmacol. Exp. Ther.* **225**: 410-415, 1983.

122. Schuurmans-Stekhoven F and Bonting SL. Transport adenosine triphosphatases: Properties and functions. *Physiol. Rev.* **61**: 2-76, 1981.

123. Schwartz A, Lindemayer GE and Allen JC. The sodium-potassium, adenosine triphosphatase: Pharmacological, physiological and biochemical aspects. *Pharmacol. Rev.* **27**: 3-134, 1975.

124. Gadsby DC. The Na K pump of cardiac cells. *Ann. Rev. Biophys. Bioeng.* **13**: 373-398, 1984.

125. Onji T and Liu M-S. Effects of alloxan-diabetes on the sodium-potassium adenosine triphosphate enzyme system in dog hearts. *Biochem. Biophys. Res. Commun.* **96**: 799-804, 1980.

126. Pierce GN and Dhalla NS. Sarcolemmal Na^+-K^+-ATPase activity in diabetic rat heart. *Am. J. Physiol.* **245**: C241-C247, 1983.

127. Ku DD and Sellers BM. Effects of streptozotocin diabetes and insulin treatment on myocardial sodium pump and contractility of the rat heart. *J. Pharmacol. Exp. Ther.* **222**: 395-400, 1982.

128. Heyliger CE, Prakash A and McNeill JH. Alterations in cardiac sarcolemmal Ca^{2+} pump activity during diabetes mellitus. *Am. J. Physiol.* **252**: H540-H544, 1987.

129. Makino N, Dhalla KS, Elimban V and Dhalla NS. Sarcolemmal Ca^{2+} transport in streptozotocin-induced diabetic cardiomyopathy in rats. *Am. J. Physiol.* **253**: E202-E207, 1987.

130. Pierce GN, Ramjiawan B, Dhalla NS and Ferrari R. Na^+-H^+ exchange in cardiac sarcolemmal vesicles isolated from diabetic rats. *Am. J. Physiol.* **258**: H255-H261, 1990.

131. Imanaga I, Kamegawa Y, Kamei R and Kuroiwa M. Cardiac sarcolemmal Na^+-K^+ adenosine triphosphatase (ATPase) activity in diabetic dog. In: Nagano M and Dhalla NS, eds. *The Diabetic Heart.* New York: Raven Press, Ltd.; 1991, p. 237-247.

132. Kjeldsen K, Braendgaard H, Sidenius P, Larsen JS and Norgaard A. Diabetes decreases Na^+-K^+ pump concentrations in skeletal muscles, heart ventricular muscle, and peripheral nerves of rat. *Diabetes* **36**: 842-848, 1987.

133. Fawzi A and McNeill JH. Effect of chronic streptozotocin-induced diabetes on [^{3}H] ouabain binding in the rat left ventricle. *Life Sci.* **36**: 1977-1981, 1985.

134. Reuter H. Calcium measurements through cardiac cell membranes. *Med. Res. Rev.* **5**: 427-440, 1985.

135. Reuter H. Exchange of calcium ions in the mammalian myocardium: Mechanisms and physiological significance. *Circ. Res.* **34**: 599-605, 1974.

136. Callewaert GL, Cleeman L and Morad M. Epinephrine enhances Ca^{2+} current-regulated Ca^{2+} release and Ca^{2+} reuptake in rat ventricular myocytes. *Proc. Natl. Acad. Sci. USA* **85**: 2009-2013, 1988.

137. Leblanc N and Hume JR. Sodium current-induced release of calcium from cardiac sarcoplasmic reticulum. *Science* **248**: 372-376, 1990.

138. Bridge JHB, Smoley JR and Spitzer KW. The relationship between charge movements associated with ICa and INa-Ca in cardiac myocytes. *Science* **248**: 376-378, 1990.

139. St Louis PJ and Sulakhe PV. Adenosine triphosphate-dependent calcium binding and accumulation by guinea-pig cardiac sarcolemma. *Can. J. Biochem.* **54**: 946-956, 1976.

140. Caroni P and Carafoli E. Regulation of Ca^{2+}-pumping ATPase of heart sarcolemma by a phosphorylation-dephosphorylation process. *J. Biol. Chem.* **256**: 9371-9373, 1981.

141. Vetter R, Hasse H and Will H. Potentiation effect of calmodulin and catalytic subunit of cyclic AMP-dependent protein kinase on ATP-dependent Ca^{2+} transport by sarcolemma. *FEBS Lett.* **148**: 326-330, 1982.

142. Borda E, Pascual J, Wald M and Sterin-Borda L. Hypersensitivity to calcium associated with an increased sarcolemmal Ca^{2+}-ATPase activity in diabetic rat heart. *Can. J. Cardiol.* **4**: 97-101, 1988.

143. Lazdunski M, Frelin C and Vigne P. The sodium/hydrogen exchange system in cardiac cells: Its biochemical and pharamcological properties and its role in regulating internal concentrations of sodium and internal pH. *J. Mol. Cell. Cardiol.* **17**: 1029-1042, 1985.

144. Pierce GN and Philipson KD. Na^+-H^+ exchange in cardiac sarcolemmal vesicles. *Biochim. Biophys. Acta* **818**: 109-116, 1985.

145. Lagadic-Gossmann D, Chesnais JM and Feuvray D. Intracellular pH regulation in papillary muscle cells from streptozotocin diabetic rats: An ion-sensitive microelectrode study. *Pflugers Arch.* **412**: 613-617, 1988.

146. Khandoudi N, Bernard M, Cozzone P and Feuvray D. Intracellular pH and the role of Na^+/H^+ exchange during ischaemia and reperfusion of normal and diabetic rat hearts. *Cardiovasc. Res.* **24**: 873-878, 1990.

147. Papahadjopoulos D, Cowden M and Kimelberg H. Role of cholesterol in membranes. Effects on phospholipid-protein interactions, membrane permeability and enzymatic activity. *Biochim. Biophys. Acta* **330**: 8-20, 1973.

148. Pierce GN, Kutryk MJB and Dhalla NS. Alterations in calcium binding and composition of the cardiac sarcolemmal membrane in chronic diabetes. *Proc. Natl. Acad. Sci. USA* **80**: 5412-5416, 1983.

149. Katz AM and Messineo FC. Lipid-membrane interactions and the pathogenesis of ischemic damage in the myocardium. *Circ. Res.* **48**: 1-16, 1981.

150. Sedlis SP, Corr PB, Sobel BE and Ahumada GG. Lysophosphatidyl-choline potentiates Ca^{2+} accumulation in rat cardiac myocytes. *Am. J. Physiol.* **244**: H32-H38, 1983.

151. Nordin C, Gilat E and Aronson RS. Delayed after depolarizations and triggered activity in ventricular muscle from rats with streptozotocin-induced diabetes. *Circ. Res.* **57**: 28-34, 1985.

152. Senges J, Brackman J, Pelzer D, Hasslackher C, Weibe E and Kubler W. Altered cardiac automaticity and conduction in experimental diabetes mellitus. *J. Mol. Cell. Cardiol.* **12**: 1341-1351, 1980.

153. Fein FS, Aronson RS, Nordin C, Miller-Green B and Sonnenblick EH. Altered myocardial response to ouabain in diabetic rats: Mechanics and electrophysiology. *J. Mol. Cell. Cardiol.* **15**: 769-776, 1983.

154. Chien KR, Reeves JP, Buja LM, Bonte F, Parkey RW and Willerson JT. Phospholipid alterations in canine ischemic myocardium. Temporal and topographical correlations with TC-99-PPi accumulation and in vitro sarcolemmal Ca^{2+} permeability defect. *Circ. Res.* **48**: 711-719, 1981.

155. Karli JN, Karikas GA, Hatzipavlou PK, Lewis GM and Moulopoulos SN. The inhibition of Na^+ and K^+-stimulated ATPase activity of rabbit and dog heart sarcolemma by lysophosphatidylcholine. *Life Sci.* **24**: 1869-1876, 1979.

156. Golfman LS, Hata T, Panagia V and Dhalla NS. Depression of cardiac Na^+-Ca^{2+} exchange by palmitoyl carnitine and lysophosphatidylcholine. *Can. J. Cardiol.* **10** (Suppl A): 75A, 1994.

157. Vecchini A, Binaglia L, Di Nardo P, Hays J-A, Panagia V and Dhalla NS. Molecular species composition of heart sarcolemmal phosphatidylcholine in diabetic cardiomyopathy. *Can. J. Cardiol.* **10** (Suppl A): 105A, 1994.

158. Crews FT. Phospholipid methylation and membrane function. In: *Phospholipids and Cellular Regulation*, Vol. 1. Kuo JF (ed). CRC Press, Boca Raton, FL, 1985, p. 131-158.

159. Panagia V, Okumura K, Makino N and Dhalla NS. Stimulation of Ca^{2+} pump in rat heart sarcolemma by

phosphatidylethanolamine N-methylation. *Biochim. Biophys. Acta* **856**: 383-387, 1986.

160. Ganguly PK, Panagia V, Okumura K and Dhalla NS. Activation of Ca^{2+}-stimulated ATPase by phospholipid N-methylation in cardiac sarcoplasmic reticulum. *Biochem. Biophys. Res. Commun.* **130**: 472-478, 1985.

161. Panagia V, Makino N, Ganguly PK and Dhalla NS. Inhibition of Na^+-Ca^{2+} exchange in heart sarcolemmal vesicles by phosphatidylethanolamine N-methylation. *Eur. J. Biochem.* **166**: 597-603, 1987.

162. Ganguly PK, Rice KM, Panagia V and Dhalla NS. Sarcolemmal phosphatidylethanolamine N-methylation in diabetic cardiomyopathy. *Circ. Res.* **55**: 504-512, 1984.

163. Panagia V, Taira Y, Ganguly PK, Tung S and Dhalla NS. Alterations in phospholipid N-methylation of cardiac subcellular membranes due to experimentally induced diabetes in rats. *J. Clin. Invest.* **86**: 777-784, 1990.

164. Frank JS, Langer GA, Nudd LM and Seraydarian K. The myocardial cell surface, its histochemistry and the effect of sialic acid and calcium removal on its structure and cellular ionic exchange. *Circ. Res.* **41**: 702-708, 1977.

165. Langer GA. The structure and function of the myocardial cell surface. *Am. J. Physiol.* **235**: H461-H468, 1978.

166. Regan TJ, Wu CF, Yeh CK, Oldewurtel HA and Haider B. Myocardial composition and function in diabetes: The effects of chronic insulin use. *Circ. Res.* **49**: 1268-1277, 1981.

167. Nagase N, Tamura Y, Kobayashi S, Saito M, Niki T, Chikamori K and Mori H. Myocardial disorders of hereditary diabetic KK mice. *J. Mol. Cell. Cardiol.* **13** (Suppl 2): 70, 1981.

168. Philipson KD, Bers DM and Nishimoto AY. The role of phospholipids in the Ca^{2+} binding of isolated cardiac sarcolemma. *J. Mol. Cell. Cardiol.* **12**: 1159-1165, 1980.

CHAPTER 7

Ketone Body Metabolism in the Diabetic Heart

John R. Forder

Introduction

Diabetes is associated with an increased incidence of heart failure that is not associated with other risk factors, such as atherosclerosis, coronary artery disease, or hypertension [1-3]. Under conditions where the disease is not well controlled, there may also be an elevation in the concentration of circulating ketone bodies. This information, coupled with the observations that isolated rat hearts are unable to sustain physiologic workloads when presented with ketone bodies as the sole energetic substrate, have led some to suggest that the myocardial dysfunction associated with diabetes could be the result of the elevation in ketone body concentration [4].

In 1938 Waters *et al.* [5] and Barnes *et al.* [6] found that in heart lung preparations the addition of ketone bodies to the perfusate resulted in their rapid uptake by the myocardium. Sixteen years later Bing noted that under *in vivo* conditions ketone bodies could account for 5-10% of the total oxygen consumption of the intact human heart [7]. It has been demonstrated that ketone bodies are utilized by the myocardium in preference to glucose or pyruvate [8-11], and in preference to free fatty acids (FFA) [10-12]. Ketone bodies may not only serve as oxidizable substrates for various tissues but also may assume the role of metabolic regulators. Under conditions where ketone bodies are present as the sole metabolic substrate [13,14], or present in very high concentrations [15] they may be deleterious to myocardial contraction; however, when present in physiologic concentrations [16] or in the presence of other substrates [17-19], they do not appear to exert such an effect.

Despite the identification of ketone bodies as endogenous substrates for myocardial energy metabolism, the study of ketone bodies as metabolic fuels for the heart has been somewhat lacking. Although the pathway by which these compounds are ultimately oxidized is well known, the modulatory effects of ketone bodies upon the pathways of intermediary energy metabolism has been the subject of relatively few investigations. This chapter will review the metabolic processes involved in the production of ketone bodies, as well as to attempt to address what is known about the inhibitory actions of these agents upon the pathways of glycolysis, glycogen synthesis, ß-oxidation, lipolysis, and the TCA cycle.

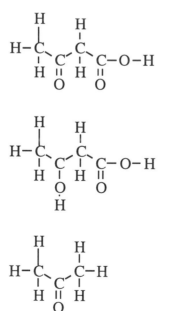

Acetoacetate

β-Hydroxybutyrate

Acetone

Figure 7.1: Chemical structure of ketone bodies.

144

Lastly, it will attempt to review what is known about the alterations that occur in the diabetic heart, where prolonged exposure to elevated ketone bodies, hyperlipidemia, and hyperglycemia may cause substantial alterations in intermediary energy metabolism.

Ketogenesis

The three compounds commonly referred to as ketone bodies are ß-hydroxybutyrate, acetoacetate, and acetone (see Figure 7.1); strictly speaking, acetone is a ketone, and not a precursor keto-alcohol. Acetone is the spontaneous breakdown product of acetoacetate -- a nonenzymatic hydrolysis -- rather than the enzymatic synthesis that form both ß-hydroxybutyrate and acetoacetate. Nevertheless, the presence of elevated acetone in the breath with its characteristic odor is taken as a clinical indication of ketosis. Both ß-hydroxybutyrate and acetoacetate are the predominant forms found in the blood.

The predominant pathway for ketone body formation occurs in the liver under conditions of high free fatty acid concentrations and low glucose oxidation; as such, their concentration is elevated during fasting, and in pathophysiologic conditions such as diabetes mellitus, following myocardial ischemia, and cancer (cachexia). The cause for ketone body synthesis under these conditions is the low concentration of oxaloacetate present in the absence of glycolytic substrate. The available oxaloacetate is utilized for gluco-neogenesis, and as a result is not available for the condensation reaction with acetyl-CoA to form citrate, which comprises the first step in the citric acid cycle. The ensuing increase in acetyl-CoA concentration drives the production of acetoacetyl-CoA via acetoacetyl-CoA thiolase (EC 2.3.1.9). Acetoacetyl-CoA condenses with another acetyl-CoA via hydroxymethylglutaryl CoA synthetase to form 3-hydroxy-3-methylglutaryl CoA. An acetyl-CoA is liberated by hydroxymethylglutaryl CoA cleavage enzyme and acetoacetate is formed. Acetoacetate is in equilibrium with ß-hydroxybutyrate via the 3-hydroxybutyrate dehydrogenase (EC 1.1.1.30). The acetoacetate to ß-hydroxybutyrate ratio is determined by the intramitochondrial NADH/NAD ratio, since this is the cofactor for the dehydrogenase.

145

Although the predominant site of ketone body synthesis is in the liver, there have been reports that pseudo-ketogenesis can occur in a number of different tissues, including the heart [20-22]. This is distinguished from the classical synthesis in that it does not require the formation of 3-hydroxymethylglutaryl CoA, but rather a reversal of the 3-oxoacid CoA transferase (EC 2.8.3.5), the enzyme that usually is involved in the metabolism of ketone bodies. It is not known if this pathway plays a significant role, although it has been suggested that it may occur *in vivo* [20].

Utilization of ketone bodies

Enzymes required for the utilization of ketone bodies include 3-hydroxybutyrate dehydrogenase (EC 1.1.1.30), 3-oxoacid CoA transferase (EC 2.8.3.5), and acetoacetyl-CoA thiolase (EC 2.3.1.9). Hearts from mice, rats, rabbits, guinea pig and dog all exhibit high activities for these enzymes, higher than the activities noted in either the gastrocnemius or the diaphragm. Guinea pig does exhibit lower activities than the other species studied thus far, but the enzyme activity pattern remains the same. In fact, of all the organs studied, the heart has one of the highest activities of these enzymes (liver has the highest activity, followed by the kidney and Harderian gland) [23].

ß-Hydroxybutyrate is metabolized in the mitochondria to acetoacetate via 3-hydroxybutyrate dehydrogenase. In most tissues, the reaction is stereospecific for the D(-)-isomer, although it has been reported that some tissue mitochondria can metabolize either isoform. Acetoacetate is converted to acetoacetyl-CoA by the enzyme 3-oxoacid CoA transferase (EC 2.8.3.5), which transfers the CoA moiety from succinyl-CoA (a TCA cycle intermediate). Acetoacetyl-CoA is subsequently cleaved via acetoacetyl-CoA thiolase (EC 2.3.1.9) in a hydrolysis reaction to yield two molecules of acetyl-CoA, which then enter the TCA cycle (see Figure 7. 2) [23].

In experiments using isolated myocyte preparations, Chen *et al.* [25] reported that the addition of lactate, octanoate, or palmitate had little, if any, effect on ß-hydroxybutyrate oxidation. However,

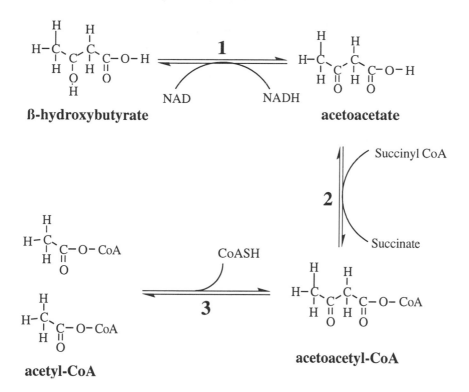

Figure 7.2: Metabolism of ketone bodies to acetyl-CoA. These reactions occur in the mitochondria, and are freely reversible. 1= 3-hydroxybutyrate dehydrogenase; 2 = 3-oxoacid-CoA transferase; 3 = acetoacetyl-CoA thiolase

ß-hydroxybutyrate oxidation was reduced by 22—28% in myocytes isolated from chronically diabetic rats, whereas the oxidation of palmitate remained similar to the controls [25].

In diabetes, there is decreased ß-hydroxybutyrate dehydrogenase enzyme activity and content [24,26-28] (see Figure 7.3), which may account for the lowered metabolism of these substrates. Interestingly, although the changes in enzyme content were reversed following insulin treatment, mitochondrial enzyme activity did not return to control levels [24,26,27]. This may be the result of alterations in mitochondrial phospholipid composition following the induction of diabetes [24,26], since the activity of the dehydrogenase is modulated by phospholipids. However, Grinblat *et al.* [28] reported no differences in mitochondrial lipid composition following the induction of diabetes, nor was mitochondrial membrane fluidity altered. These results are consistent with those of Vidal *et al.* [26], who reported that the decrease in dehydrogenase activity was due to a decrease in the amount of enzyme in the inner mitochondrial membrane rather than a modification of mitochondrial lipid composition. It remains to be determined, however, if administration of insulin alters the mitochondrial lipid composition in diabetic heart, which might explain the temporal separation between the recovery of enzyme content and the observed enzyme activity.

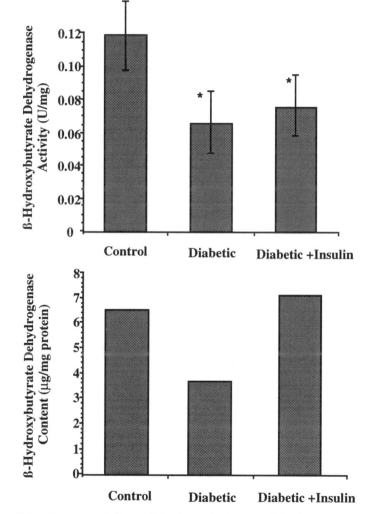

Figure 7.3: Top panel shows ß-hydroxybutyrate dehydrogenase activity from mitochondria isolated from control, diabetic, and insulin-treated diabetic rat hearts. * = significantly different from control. Bottom panel shows enzyme content from pooled samples, determined immunohistochemically for the same three groups. Data from Kante *et al.* [24].

In addition to the changes in 3-hydroxybutyrate dehydrogenase activity, the activity of the myocardial 3-oxoacid CoA transferase is also reduced approximately 50% in rats following three months of streptozocin-induced diabetes, while the activity of the myocardial acetoacetyl-CoA thiolase was unaffected [28].

Inhibition of glycolysis

Ketone bodies have been reported to decrease glucose uptake, presumably through an inhibition of glycolysis at hexokinase [29,30], phosphofructokinase [29] and pyruvate dehydrogenase [10,31-33]. The presence of ketone bodies has also been reported to stimulate glycogen synthesis [29,34-36].

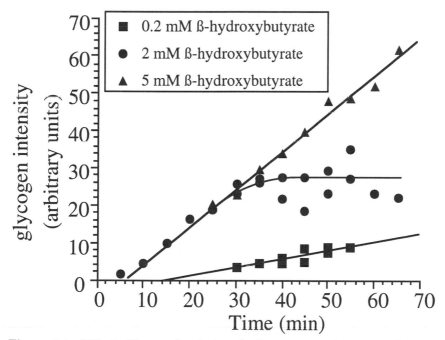

Figure 7.4: Effect of increasing ketone body concentration upon glycogen synthesis in the intact rat heart. Experiments were performed on isolated rat hearts perfused with [1-^{13}C]glucose and ß-hydroxybutyrate (n=4 for each concentration). Glycogen intensity is proportional to myocardial glycogen concentration, and is plotted as a function of time following presentation of the ^{13}C-labeled glucose.

Recent experiments from our laboratory using isolated rat hearts perfused with buffer containing [1-^{13}C]glucose and increasing concentrations of ß-hydroxybutyrate have demonstrated a dose dependent increase in glycogen synthesis (see Figure 7.4). Although the concentration dependent increase in myocardial glycogen synthesis observed with ketone bodies has been in hearts from control animals [29,34-36], they may also play a role in the increased glycogen content of the myocardium in diabetes. This is discussed in more detail in Chapter 8.

Lactate oxidation in the heart is also inhibited by ß-hydroxybutyrate, and is probably due to diminished oxidation of pyruvate as a result of greater conversion of pyruvate dehydrogenase (PDH) from the active to inactive form [10,31-33]. Increased acetyl-CoA/CoA ratio in the mitochondria due to enhanced ketone utilization has been associated with increased phosphorylation of PDH kinase and the subsequent inactivation of PDH [32,33]. Recent experiments using isolated rat hearts perfused with a physiologic mixture of palmitate (0.7mM), glucose (5mM), and increasing concentrations of ß-hydroxybutyrate (0-5mM) showed glucose to be maximally inhibited (from 36% to 13%) at a ß-hydroxybutyrate concentration as low as 0.2mM (see Figure 7.5) [37]. To the author's knowledge, the inhibitory effects of ketone bodies upon glycolysis and glucose oxidation have not been studied in the diabetic heart -- this remains a rich area for future work.

Inhibition of ß-oxidation

Ketone bodies are known to be oxidized by the heart in preference to fatty acids, resulting in reduced fatty acid uptake and oxidation (see Figure 7.5) [11,12,37-40]. In contrast to the decreased palmitate oxidation, octanoate oxidation in isolated myocytes was only slightly inhibited by ß-hydroxybutyrate [25], suggesting that inhibition of fatty acid oxidation occurs at the mitochondrial transport step. However, Forsey et al. [11] reported that both palmitate and octanoate oxidation were inhibited in isolated rat hearts perfused with either ß-hydroxybutyrate (5mM) or acetoacetate (5mM). As a result, inhibition of fatty acid oxidation by ketone bodies may involve not only the oxidation step, but also the carnitine mediated transfer of fatty acids into the mitochondria. This was supported by the findings of Menahan and Hron [38], where there was a dramatic increase in the long chain fatty acylcarnitine/carnitine ratio in hearts perfused with acetoacetate in addition to palmitate. In addition, acetoacetyl-CoA has also been reported to inhibit the general acyl-CoA dehydrogenase from pig liver [40], and may play a role in the decreased oxidation of fatty acids that accompanies an elevation in the ketone body concentration.

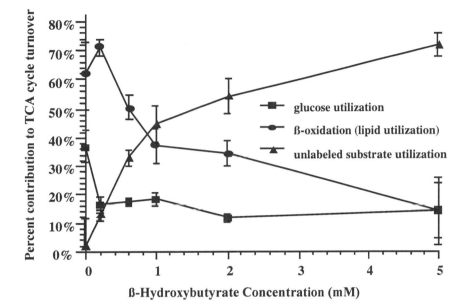

Figure 7.5 Effect of ketone body concentration upon glucose and palmitate oxidation in the isolated rat heart. Graph shows the contribution of both glucose and palmitate to the TCA cycle in the presence of increasing concentrations of ß-hydroxybutyrate (n=4-6 at each concentration). Inhibition of palmitate oxidation occurs at a higher concentration of ß-hydroxybutyrate than the inhibition of glucose oxidation. Unlabeled substrate utilization corresponds to ß-hydroxybutyrate oxidation.

In ventricular myocytes isolated from diabetic animals, the concentration-dependent inhibition of palmitate oxidation by ß-hydroxybutyrate was unchanged compared to myocytes isolated from control animals [41]. Thus the inhibition of ß-oxidation (or perhaps carnitine acyltransferase) by ketone bodies remains unaffected in the diabetic heart, despite a decrease in the enzymatic machinery required to metabolize ketone bodies (see Figure 7.3) for energy production [24,26-28].

Effects on lipolysis

Larsen *et al.* [41], using isolated calcium-tolerant ventricular myocytes from normal and diabetic rats (100mg/kg streptozocin, 3days), examined the effect of oleate (0.3 and 1.2 mM) and the combined effect of ß-hydroxybutyrate (4 and 8 mM) and acetoacetate (1 and 2 mM) on lipolytic rates. Glycerol output was used as an index of lipolysis. Myocytes from diabetic rats had higher lipolytic rates than normal myocytes. In control myocytes, addition of oleate (1.2 mM) did not affect basal lipolysis; whereas, the addition of oleate to diabetic myocytes inhibited basal rates of lipolysis by 41%. Despite the inhibition by oleate, lipolysis was still higher in diabetic myocytes than in normal myocytes incubated in the absence of oleate. Ketone bodies increased both basal and isoproterenol-stimulated lipolysis in normal myocytes. However in diabetic myocytes ketone bodies produced a only modest stimulation of basal lipolysis and had no effect on isoproterenol stimulated rates of lipolysis.

In contrast, Hron *et al.* [42] and Lammerant *et al.* [43] reported that ketone bodies inhibited myocardial lipolysis in the isolated perfused rat heart and the intact dog, respectively. It is yet to be determined if the stimulation of lipolysis noted by Larsen *et al.* [41] is the result of the myocyte isolation or cell perfusion conditions, or whether the reported inhibition of myocardial lipolysis [42,43] is due to the effect of ketone bodies upon the cardioadipocytes known to be present in the intact myocardium [41]. Regardless, the observed myocardial accumulation of triglycerides observed in diabetic ketosis is more likely due to enhancement of synthesis [40] resulting from the elevation in acetoacetyl-CoA and the subsequent high circulating levels of exogenous fatty acids and alterations in the CoA-carnitine relationship [44], rather than through an inhibition of lipolysis by the elevation in ketone body concentration [41].

152

Inhibition of the TCA cycle

Despite the predilection of cardiac tissue for ketone body fuels, it has been shown that the isolated, working heart demonstrates impaired function when provided ketone bodies in the absence of other metabolic substrates [13,14,18,22,45]. Though it has been shown that this functional impairment does not occur when ketone bodies are supplemented with other metabolic fuels [11,12,16-19,22,39,46-49], it has been suggested that the observed functional deficit may have implications in the etiology of heart failure in ketotic states. As ketosis has been shown to occur in a variety of physiologic and pathophysiologic conditions, including diabetes and malignant cachexia, further experiments using ketone bodies in the presence of other metabolic substrates have been warranted, to attempt to further our knowledge of the effect of ketone bodies on cardiac viability. Although ketone bodies can make a major contribution to the energy supply of the working heart, a second substrate such as glucose is apparently needed to meet the energy requirements for the pump function at physiological pressures [13,14,18,45]. In order to be oxidized, acetoacetate has to be converted to acetyl-CoA. It has been suggested by Taegtmeyer [13] that the rates of acetyl-CoA formation from acetoacetate may be too low under conditions of high myocardial work, presumably because the capacity of the thiolase reaction is the step limiting acetoacetate utilization [23]. The limited rate of acetyl-CoA formation from acetoacetate appears to be sufficient for the heart perfused by the Langendorff technique [9], but not for the working hearts where at physiological pressure oxygen consumption is 2.5 times higher. However, earlier experiments by Garland and Randle [10], as well as reports from Taegtmeyer *et al.* [13], Russell *et al.* [45] and Menahan *et al.* [38] have all shown that the acetyl-CoA concentration increases in hearts perfused with ketone bodies. This suggests that still another mechanism may be responsible for the inability of ketone bodies to support the working heart when present as the sole metabolic substrate [13,50].

Reports from several laboratories have suggested that inhibition of the 2-oxoglutarate dehydrogenase, either as a result of decreased concentration of intramitochondrial CoASH [13,14,45] or an increase in the NADH/NAD ratio [19,46], may be responsible for the inability of ketone bodies to maintain physiologic work when present as the sole substrate for myocardial energy metabolism. Consistent with inhibition of this enzyme, provision of ketone bodies as metabolic substrates have been associated with elevations in myocardial aconitate, α-ketoglutarate, glutamate, and malate concentrations, as well as decreases in free CoASH, succinyl-CoA, fumarate, and oxaloacetate [13,14,18,22,45]. Forsey et al. [11], using a open chest dog preparation, examined the arterio-venous differences of a number of substrates as the animal was infused with increasing concentrations of ketone bodies. In addition to an inhibition of myocardial lactate, glucose, and fatty acid extraction, subsequent freeze-clamping and acid extraction of the myocardium revealed increased pool sizes of glutamate and citrate, and decreased concentration of succinyl-CoA. Consistent with previous observations made by Taegtmeyer in the isolated perfused rat heart [13], the authors concluded that elevation of ketone bodies *in vivo* also inhibited the 2-oxoglutarate dehydrogenase.

^{13}C-NMR spectroscopy is able to detect chemical species in the 100 micromolar to millimolar range. As a result, most of the TCA cycle intermediates are below the level of detection using this technique. Glutamate, however, is present in sufficient quantity for detection by NMR, and has the added advantage of being in rapid exchange equilibrium with α-ketoglutarate. Therefore, it has been suggested that the rate of incorporation of a ^{13}C label from a metabolic substrate into the glutamate pool reflects TCA cycle turnover [58,63,64]. Moreover, if a substrate is administered which yields acetyl CoA labeled in the 2-carbon, then following the condensation reaction with oxaloacetate, the label appears in the 4-carbon position of citrate, and subsequently α-ketoglutarate and glutamate. On subsequent turns of the TCA cycle, the label in the 4-carbon position of α-ketoglutarate (and therefore, by necessity glutamate) is randomized into the 2 and 3 carbon positions of fumarate, due to the symmetry of the molecule. Following the next condensation reaction, the 2 and 3 carbon labeled oxaloacetate yields 2 and 3 carbon labeled α-ketoglutarate (in combination with label in the 4-carbon position arising from the incoming 2-carbon labeled acetyl CoA) which exchanges again with glutamate. As a

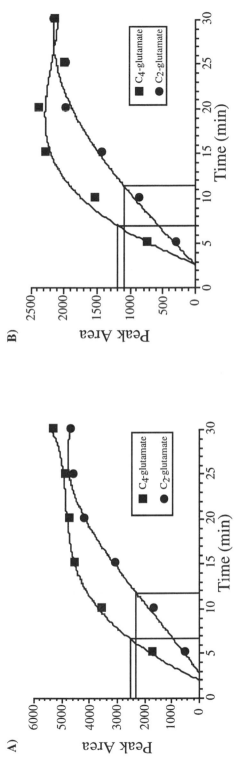

Figure 7.6: Comparison of glutamate labeling rates following perfusion with either A) [4-¹³C]β-hydroxybutyrate plus unlabeled glucose, or B) [1-¹³C]glucose alone. ¹³C NMR spectra (uncorrected for saturation or nuclear Overhauser enhancement) are shown from representative experiments. *Note the increased peak area in the heart perfused with β-hydroxybutyrate, reflecting the increased glutamate pool. The ratio of the time for half maximal labeling of the C₄-glutamate to the time for half maximal labeling of the C₂-glutamate reflects TCA cycle flux, and is independent of glutamate pool size [59]. If inhibition of 2-oxoglutarate dehydrogenase had occurred due to the presence of β-hydroxybutyrate, this should be reflected by changes in the ratio of labeling rates.*

155

result, these experiments not only yield information regarding the rate of TCA cycle turnover, but also provide an index of the entry of substrates into TCA cycle at locations other than acetyl-CoA (so-called anaplerotic reactions). For example, under conditions of increased anaplerosis, the labeling of the C_3 and C_2 glutamate at steady state should be less than the labeling of the C_4 glutamate, due to dilution at sites following α-ketoglutarate in the TCA cycle. Experiments performed in our laboratory using isolated rat hearts perfused with either [4-^{13}C]ß-hydroxybutyrate (which produces 2-^{13}C-acetyl-CoA) or [1-^{13}C]glucose (which also produces 2-^{13}C-acetyl-CoA) showed no differences between either the absolute rates of label incorporation into the C_4 and C_3 of glutamate, or the ratio of the rates of ^{13}C incorporation into the C_3 and C_4 positions of glutamate (see Figure 7.6). Using a network model of linear differential equations to estimate the absolute flux through a number of biochemical pathways (TCA cycle, malate-aspartate shuttle, malic enzyme, proteolysis, and α-glycerol phosphate shuttle) from the ^{13}C NMR data combined with oxygen consumption measurements, the flux through anaplerotic pathways was not elevated during perfusion with ß-hydroxybutyrate, nor was the actual TCA cycle flux rate altered [64]. While we have observed an increase in glutamate concentration at higher ß-hydroxybutyrate concentrations, consistent with inhibition of 2-oxoglutarate dehydrogenase, the energy deficit caused by such a blockade would require increased anaplerosis to maintain ATP production [13,14,18,22]. We have shown that this does not occur over the time course (and with the temporal resolution) of these experiments.

We did not observe any decrement in contractile function, although this would not be expected due to 1) the presence of glucose in the ß-hydroxybutyrate-perfused heart, and 2) the use of the isovolumic Langendorff preparation. The demonstration of a lack of functional change with increasing ß-hydroxybutyrate concentrations in our studies is consistent with previous experiments which have examined the effect of increasing ketone body concentration on heart function in the presence of other metabolic fuels [11,12,16-19,22,39,46-49].

Additionally, the method of heart preparation utilized by Taegtmeyer differs from that used in our experiments. The working heart is made to perfuse its own coronary circulation, so a mild decrease in function would lead to lowered coronary flows, and subsequent hypoxia and worsening failure. The modified Langendorff preparation can undergo an early period of mildly decreased function without sacrificing coronary perfusion, and thus may be better suited to survive a transient functional deficit. Assuming that there exists a functional deficit in both heart preparations which is transient and reversible, there may not be any steady-state impairment on function on the Langendorff preparation, whereas the working heart preparation might fail.

Thus, one can imagine the existence of a transient inhibition of 2-oxoglutarate dehydrogenase, perhaps due to a deficiency in intra-mitochondrial CoASH. This deficit in energy production may cause a transient increase in anaplerosis, and after a sufficient concentration of α-ketoglutarate has accumulated, the blockade is relieved, TCA cycle flux returns to normal and anaplerosis drops back down to pre-stress levels, and is thus unchanged at steady-state.

Summary

Further research remains to be done to fully characterize the dramatic and diverse metabolic alterations that occur in the diabetic heart subjected to elevated ketone body concentrations. It is apparent that ketone bodies can inhibit glycolysis and glucose oxidation by the heart even at low concentrations. They stimulate glycogen synthesis, and have been reported to inhibit both hexokinase and phosphofructokinase. Pyruvate dehydrogenase is also inhibited, preventing carbon units from glucose from entering the TCA cycle. Furthermore, they can inhibit fatty acid oxidation at both physiologic concentrations as well as pathophysiologic concentrations. It remains to be determined whether the inhibition of fatty acid oxidation by ketone bodies occurs at the level of transport into the mitochondria via carnitine acyltransferase, or whether there is a direct inhibitory effect upon ß-oxidation. With reference to lipolysis, it appears that ketone bodies may have different effects on ventricular myocytes (stimulatory) versus intact cardiac preparations that may contain cardioadipocytes (inhibitory). Much work remains to be done with respect to the effects of ketone bodies upon the TCA cycle, and the elucidation of the mechanisms by which they cause dramatic alterations in the concentrations of various TCA cycle intermediates. The observation that their metabolism may be altered in the diabetic heart, coupled with the elevated concentration in blood often seen in diabetics, makes this area a particularly important one for future research.

Acknowledgments

This work was supported by a grant from the American Heart Association, with funds provided in part by the AHA, Maryland Affiliate.

References

1. Kannel WB, Hjortland M and Castelli WP. Role of diabetes in congestive heart failure: The Framingham Study. *Am. J. Cardiol.* **34**: 29-34, 1974.

2. Kannel WB and McGee DL. Diabetes and cardiovascular risk factors: The Framingham study. *Circulation* **59**: 8-13, 1979.

3. Kannel WB and McGee DL. Diabetes and cardiovascular disease: The Framingham study. *JAMA* **241**: 2035-2038, 1979.

4. Taegtmeyer H. Defective energy metabolism of the heart in diabetes. *Lancet* **1**: 139-141, 1985.

5. Waters ET, Fletcher JP and Mirsky IA. The relation between carbohydrate and ß-hydroxybutyric acid utilization by the heart-lung preparation. *Am. J. Physiol.* **122**: 542-546, 1938.

6. Barnes RH, MacKay EM, Moe GK and Visscher MB. The utilization of hydroxybutyric acid by the isolated mammalian heart and lung. *Am. J. Physiol.* **122**: 272-279, 1938.

7. Bing RJ, Siegel A, Unger I and Gilbert M. Metabolism of the human heart. II. Studies on fat, ketone and amino acid metabolism. *Am. J. Med.* **16**: 540-615, 1954.

8. Hall LM. Preferential oxidation of acetoacetate by the perfused heart. *Biochem. Biophys. Res. Comm.* **6**: 177-179, 1961.

9. Williamson JR and Krebs HA. Acetoacetate as fuel of respiration in the perfused rat heart. *Biochem. J.* **80**: 540-547, 1961.

10. Garland PB, Newsholme EA and Randle PJ. Regulation of glucose uptake by muscle. 9: Effects of fatty acids, ketone bodies and of alloxan-diabetes and starvation, on pyruvate metabolism and on lactate/pyruvate and l-glycerol 3-phosphate/dihydroxyacetone phosphate concentration ratios in rat heart and rat diaphragm muscles. *Biochem. J.* **93**: 664-678, 1964.

11. Forsey RG, Reid K and Brosnan JT. Competition between fatty acids and carbohydrate or ketone bodies as metabolic fuels for the isolated perfused heart. *Can J Physiol Pharmacol* **65**: 401-6, 1987.

12. Little JR, Goto M and Spitzer JJ. Effect of ketones on metabolism of free fatty acids by dog myocardium and skeletal muscle in vivo. *Am. J. Physiol.* **219**: 1458-1463, 1970.

13. Taegtmeyer H. On the inability of ketone bodies to serve as the only energy providing substrate for rat heart at physiological work load. *Basic Res Cardiol* **78**: 435-450, 1983.

14. Russell RR and Taegtmeyer H. Changes in citric acid cycle flux and anaplerosis antedate the functional decline in isolated rat hearts utilizing acetoacetate. *J. Clin. Invest.* **87**: 384-390, 1991.

15. Zimmerman ANE, Meijler FL and Hulsmann WC. The inhibitory effect of acetoacetate on myocardial contraction. *Lancet* **2**: 757-758, 1962.

16. Bassenge E, Wendt VE, Schollmeyer P, Blumchen G, Gudbjamason S and Bing RJ. Effect of ketone bodies on cardiac metabolism. *Am. J. Physiol.* **208**: 162-168, 1965.

17. Breuer J, Chung KJ, Pesonen E, Haas RH, Guth BD, Sahn DJ and Hesselink JR. Ketone bodies maintain normal cardiac function and myocardial high energy phosphates during

insulin-induced hypoglycemia in vivo. *Basic Res. Cardiol.* **84**: 510-23, 1989.

18. Russell RRd and Taegtmeyer H. Pyruvate carboxylation prevents the decline in contractile function of rat hearts oxidizing acetoacetate. *Am. J. Physiol.* 1991.

19. Kim DK, Heineman FW and Balaban RS. Effects of ß-hydroxybutyrate on oxidative metabolism and phosphorylation potential in canine heart in vivo. *Am. J. Physiol.* **260**: H1767-H1773, 1991.

20. Fink G, Desrochers S, Des RC, Garneau M, David F, Daloze T, Landau BR and Brunengraber H. Pseudoketogenesis in the perfused rat heart. *J. Biol. Chem.* **263**: 18036-42, 1988.

21. LaNoue K, Nicklas WJ and Williamson JR. Control of citric acid cycle activity in rat heart mitochondria. *J. Biol. Chem.* **245**: 102-111, 1970.

22. Russell RR, Mommessin JI and Taegtmeyer H. Propionyl-L-carnitine-mediated improvement in contractile function of rat hearts oxidizing acetoacetate. *Am. J. Physiol.* **268**: H441-H447, 1995.

23. Williamson DH, Bates MW, Page MA and Krebs HA. Activities of enzymes involved in acetoacetate utilization in adult mammalian tissues. *Biochem. J.* **121**: 41-47, 1971.

24. Kante A, Malki MC, Coquard C and Latruffe N. Metabolic control of the expression of mitochondrial D-beta-hydroxybutyrate dehydrogenase, a ketone body converting enzyme. *Biochim. Biophys. Acta* **1033**: 291-297, 1990.

25. Chen V, Wagner G and Spitzer JJ. Regulation of substrate oxidation in isolated myocardial cells by ß-hydroxybutyrate. *Horm. Metab. Res.* **16**: 243-247, 1984.

26. Vidal JC, McIntyre JO, Churchill P, Andrew JA, Pehuet M and Fleischer S. Influence of diabetes on rat liver mitochondria: decreased unsaturation of phospholipid and D-beta-hydroxybutyrate dehydrogenase activity. *Arch. Biochem. Biophys.* **224**: 643-658, 1983.

27. Churchill P, McIntyre JO, Vidal JC and Fleischer S. Basis for decreased D-beta-hydroxybutyrate dehydrogenase activity in

liver mitochondria from diabetic rats. *Arch. Biochem. Biophys.* **224**: 659-670, 1983.

28. Grinblat L, Pacheco BnL and Stoppani AO. Decreased rate of ketone-body oxidation and decreased activity of D-3-hydroxybutyrate dehydrogenase and succinyl-CoA:3-oxo-acid CoA-transferase in heart mitochondria of diabetic rats. *Biochem. J.* **240**: 49-56, 1986.

29. Newsholme EA, Randle PJ and Manchester KL. Inhibition of the phosphofructoskinase reaction in perfused rat heart by respiration of ketone bodies, fatty acids and pyruvate. *Nature* **193**: 270-271, 1962.

30. Morgan HE, Randle PJ and Regen DM. Regulation of glucose uptake by muscle. 3. The effects of insulin, anoxia, salicylate and 2:4-dinitrophenol on membrane transport and intracellular phosphorylation of glucose in the isolated rat heart. *Biochem. J.* **73**: 573-579, 1959.

31. Garland PB and Randle PJ. Regulation of glucose uptake by muscle. 10: Effects of alloxan-diabetes, starvation, hypophysectomy and adrenalectomy and of fatty acids, ketone bodies and pyruvate, on the glycerol output and concentrations of free fatty acids, long chain fatty acyl-coenzyme A, glycerol phosphate and citrate-cycle intermediates in rat heart and diaphragm muscles. *Biochem. J.* **93**: 678-687, 1964.

32. Kerby AL, Randle PJ, Cooper RH, Whitehouse S, Pask HT and Denton RM. Regulation of pyruvate dehydrogenase in rat heart: Mechanism of regulation of properties of dephosphorylated and phosphorylated enzymes by oxidation of fatty acids and ketone bodies and of effects of diabetes: role of coenzyme A, acetyl-coenzyme A, and reduced and oxidized nicotinamide adenine dinucleotide. *Biochem. J.* **154**: 327-348, 1976.

33. Kerby AL, Radcliff PM and Randle PJ. Diabetes and the control of pyruvate dehydrogenase in rat heart mitochondria by concentration ratios of adenosine triphosphate/adenosine diphosphate, of reduced/oxidized nicotinamide-adenine dinucleotide and of acetyl-coenzyme A/coenzyme A. *Biochem. J.* **64**: 509-519, 1977.

34. Laughlin M, Taylor J, Chesnick AS and Balaban RS. Nonglucose substrates increase glycogen synthesis in vivo in dog heart. *Am. J. Physiol.* **267**: H217-H223, 1994.

35. Forder JR, Chatham JC and Glickson JD. Alteration of myocardial metabolism in theisolated perfused rat heart by ß-hydroxybutyrate: determination by ^{13}C, [13]P and ^{1}H NMR spectroscopy, *10th Annual meeting of the Society of Magnetic Resonance in Medicine*, 1; 69. San Fransisco, 1991

36. Forder JR, Chatham JC and Glickson JD. Myocardial glucose metabolism is altered in the rat heart by ß-hydroxybutyrate: detection by ^{1}H-, ^{13}C- and ^{31}P-NMR spectroscopy. *J. Mol. Cell. Cardiol.* **24** (Suppl. 1): S.83, 1992.

37. Schulman DA, Chatham JC and Forder JR. Effect of D-ß-hydroxybutyrate upon fatty acid and glucose oxidation in the isolated rat heart: Assessment using ^{13}C-NMR spectroscopy. *FASEB J.* **9**: A879, 1995.

38. Olson RE. Effect of pyruvate and acetoacetate on the metabolism of fatty acids by the perfused rat heart. *Nature (London)* **195**: 597-599, 1962.

39. Menahan L and Hron W. Regulation of acetoacetyl-CoA in isolated perfused rat hearts. *Eur. J. Biochem.* **119**: 295-299, 1981.

40. Vanoverschelde JJ, Wijns W, Kolanowski J, Bol A, Decoster PM, Michel C, Cogneau M, Heyndrickx GR, Essamri B and Melin JA. Competition between palmitate and ketone bodies as fuels for the heart: study with positron emission tomography. *Am. J. Physiol.* **264**: H701-H707, 1993.

41. Paulson DJ and Crass MF. Endogenous triacylglycerol metabolism in diabetic heart. *Am. J. Physiol.* **242**: H1084-H1094, 1982.

42. Larsen TS and Severson DL. Influence of exogenous fatty acids and ketone bodies on rates of lipolysis in isolated ventricular myocytes from normal and diabetic rats. *Can. J. Physiol. Pharmacol.* **68**: 1177-82, 1990.

43. Hron WT, Menahan LA and Lech JJ. Inhibition of hormonal stimulation of lipolysis in perfused rat heart by ketone bodies. *J. Mol. Cell. Cardiol.* **10**: 161-174, 1978.

44. Lammerant J, Huynh–Thu T and Kolanowski J. Stabilization of left ventricular function with D(-)3-hydroxybutyrate after coronary occlusion in the intact dog. *J. Mol. Cell. Cardiol.* **20**: 579-583, 1988.

45. Lopaschuk GD and Tsang H. Metabolism of palmitate in isolated working hearts from spontaneously diabetic "BB" Wistar rats. *Circ. Res.* **61**: 853-858, 1987.

46. Russell RRd and Taegtmeyer H. Coenzyme A sequestration in rat hearts oxidizing ketone bodies. *J Clin Invest* **89**: 968-73, 1992.

47. Breuer J, Chung KJ, Pesonen E, Haas RH, Guth BD, Sahn DJ and Hesselink JR. Cardiac function, substrate utilization, and myocardial energy metabolism studied with 31-P NMR spectroscopy during acute hypoglycemia and hyperketonemia. *Pediatr. Res.* **26**: 536-42, 1989.

48. Sultan AMN. D-3-hydroxybutyrate metabolism in the perfused rat heart. *Mol. Cell. Biochem.* **79**: 113-8, 1988.

49. Sultan AM. The effect of fasting on D-3-hydroxybutyrate metabolism in the perfused rat heart. *Mol. Cell. Biochem.* **93**: 107-18, 1990.

50. Sultan AM. Effects of diabetes and insulin on ketone bodies metabolism in heart. *Mol. Cell. Biochem.* **110**: 17-23, 1992.

51. Taegtmeyer H, Hems R and Krebs HA. Utilization of energy-providing substrates in the isolated rat heart. *Biochem. J.* **186**: 701-711, 1980.

52. Bailey IA, Gadian DG, Matthews PM, Radda GK and Seeley PJ. Studies of metabolism in the isolated perfused rat heart using ^{13}C NMR. *FEBS Lett.* **123**: 315-318, 1981.

53. Malloy CR, Sherry AD and Jeffery FMH. Carbon flux through citric acid cycle pathways in perfused heart by ^{13}C NMR spectroscopy. *FEBS Lett.* **212**: 58-62, 1987.

54. Malloy CR, Sherry AD and Jeffrey FMH. Evaluation of carbon flux and substrate selection through alternate pathways involving the citric acid cycle of the heart by ^{13}C NMR spectroscopy. *J. Biol. Chem.* **263**: 6964-6971, 1988.

55. Malloy CR, Thompson JR, Jeffrey FMH and Sherry AD. Contribution of exogenous substrates to acetyl coenzyme A: measurement by ^{13}C NMR under non-steady state conditions. *Biochemistry* **29**: 6756-6761, 1990.

56. Malloy CR, Sherry AD and Jeffrey FMH. Analysis of tricarboxylic acid cycle of the heart using ^{13}C isotope isomers. *Am. J. Physiol.* **259**: H987-H995, 1990.

57. Weiss RG, Chacko VP, Glickson JD and Gerstenblith G. Comparative ^{13}C and ^{31}P NMR assessment of altered metabolism during graded reductions in coronary flow in intact rat hearts. *Proc. Natl. Acad. Sci. USA* **86**: 6426-6430., 1989.

58. Weiss RG, Chacko VP and Gerstenblith G. Fatty acid regulation of glucose metabolism in the intact beating rat heart assessed by carbon-13 NMR spectroscopy: the critical role of pyruvate dehydrogenase. *J Mol Cell Cardiol* **21**: 469-478, 1989.

59. Weiss RG, Gloth ST, Kalil-Filho R, Chacko VP, Stern MD and Gerstenblith G. Indexing tricarboxylic acid cycle flux in intact hearts by carbon-13 nuclear magnetic resonance. *Circ. Res.* **70**: 392-408, 1992.

60. Chatham JC and Forder JR. A ^{13}C-NMR study of glucose oxidation in the intact functioning rat heart following diabetes-induced cardiomyopathy. *J. Mol. Cell. Cardiol.* **25**: 1203-1213, 1993.

61. Robitaille PML, Rath DP, Abduljalil AM, Odonnell JM, Jiang ZC, Zhang HZ and Hamlin RL. Dynamic ^{13}C NMR analysis of oxidative metabolism in the in vivo canine myocardium. *J. Biol. Chem.* **268**: 26296-26301, 1993.

62. Rothman DL, Behar KL, Hetherington HP, Den Hollander JA, Bendall MR, Petroff OAC and Shulman RG. ^{1}H observe/^{13}C decouple spectroscopic measurements of lactate and glutamate in the rat brain in vivo. *Proc. Natl. Acad. Sci. USA* **82**: 1633-1637, 1985.

63. Reo NV, Siegfried BA and Ackerman JJH. Direct observation of glycogenesis and glucagon stimulated glycogenolysis in the rat liver in vivo by high field carbon-13 surface coil NMR. *J. Biol. Chem.* **259**: 13664-13667, 1984.

164

64. Chance EM, Seeholzer SH, Kobayashi K and Williamson JR. Mathematical analysis of isotope labeling in the citric acid cycle with applications to ^{13}C NMR studies in perfused rat hearts. *J. Biol. Chem.* **258**: 13785-13794, 1983.

65. Chatham JC, Forder JR, Glickson JD and Chance EM. Calculation of absolute metabolic flux and the elucidation of the pathways of glutamate labeling in perfused rat heart by ^{13}C NMR spectroscopy and nonlinear least squares analysis. *J. Biol. Chem.* **270**: 7999-8008, 1995.

CHAPTER 8

Cardiac Glycogen Metabolism in Diabetes

Maren R. Laughlin

Introduction

Glucose metabolism is severely depressed in the hearts of diabetic animals due to reduced glucose uptake, reduced glycolytic activity, reduced pyruvate oxidation and reduced rates of glycogen storage [1-12]. This chapter will discuss the abnormalities of glycogen metabolism that characterize the diabetic heart. (Chapter 9 addresses the effect of diabetes on other aspects of glucose metabolism.)

Glycogen is mobilized for use in the glycolytic pathway to produce cytosolic ATP during brief periods of extreme stress such as anoxia [13], and during the increased work of heavy exercise [14-16]. Its metabolism is altered in all models of experimental diabetes that have been studied, including short-term (2-4 days) or long-term (4 weeks to several months) hypoinsulinemia caused by alloxan or streptozotocin injection [1,4,7,17] and a genetic model of spontaneous diabetes (BB/W rats) [5].

In many tissues of diabetic animals, the altered glucose metabolism either does not affect glycogen concentration, or tends to reduce it. Glycogen concentration is unchanged in gastrocnemius or plantaris muscle of diabetic rats, but in soleus, made predominantly of slow-twitch fibers, glycogen is slightly lowered [18-20]. Liver glycogen is similarly reduced from 280 µmol/g wet wt to about 80 in rats 3 weeks after being given 150 mg/kg streptozotocin and this reduction is dose-dependent [19]. However, in all animal models of diabetes the amount of glycogen stored in heart is increased compared to non-diabetic controls. Glycogen tripled to 40 µmol/g wet wt in rat heart after 3-4 weeks of streptozotocin-induced diabetes [19], and reached 70.3 µmol/g wet wt after 12 weeks of diabetes [17]. Myocardial glycogen concentration correlates with the duration and severity of the diabetic state, and is loosely associated with elevated blood glucose levels, but not with heart weight, plasma free fatty acids, triglycerides, or ketone bodies [1,19]. Ultrastructure studies of cardiomyocytes from both acute and chronic diabetic rat models show large deposits of dense glycogen granules. These are invariably clustered near the mitochondria which are swollen and distorted, and are accompanied by lipid droplets [21-24].

The outside of the spherical glycogen α-particle found in heart (10^7 daltons, 20 nm diameter, [25,26]) is strongly associated with a variety of proteins. The majority consist of the enzymes that directly metabolize glycogen (glycogen synthase, glycogen phosphorylase, branching and debranching enzymes) and the regulatory protein phosphatases and kinases that activate and inactivate them. Glycogen synthase (GS) activity is rate-limiting in the synthetic direction, and creates $\alpha-[1,4]$linkages between the glucose of uridine diphosphoglucose (UDPG) and the growing ends of the glucosyl chains on the outside of the particle. Glycogen phosphorylase (GP) is similarly rate-limiting for glycogen breakdown, and uses inorganic phosphate (P_i) to cleave glucose 1-phosphate (G1P) from the glucosyl chains. In addition, branching and debranching enzymes are necessary to metabolize glycogen at the $\alpha-[1,6]$ branch points between glucosyl chains, but these are thought to exist in concentrations too high to be rate-limiting [27]. Figure 8.1 is a schematic of glycogen metabolism in the heart. GS and GP are controlled both by covalent modification of the protein by protein kinases and phosphatases (addition or subtraction of phosphate groups to specific serine residues) and allosteric binding of small molecules to regulatory domains [27,28].

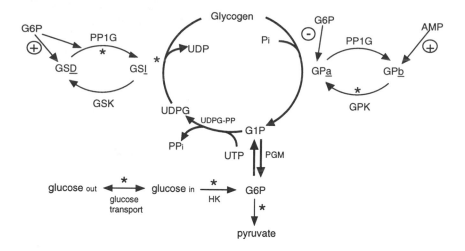

Figure 8.1: A schematic of glycogen metabolism in the heart, with the sites affected by diabetes marked with an asterisk. Abbreviations are glucose 6-phosphate (G6P); glucose 1-phosphate (G1P); uridine diphosphoglucose (UDPG); pyrophosphate (PP$_i$); inorganic phosphate (P$_i$); phosphoglucomutase (PGM); hexokinase (HK); UDP-glucose pyrophosphorylase (UDPG-PP); glycogen synthase (GS); glycogen phosphorylase (GP); phosphoprotein phosphatase (PP1G); glycogen synthase kinases (GSK); glycogen phosphorylase kinase (GPK). GS exists in both active (GS<u>i</u>) and inactive forms (GS<u>d</u>) which are interconverted by GSK and PP1G. GS<u>d</u> can also be activated by allosteric binding of G6P, which then makes it a better substrate for activation by PP1G. GP exists as the active, AMP-independent form (GP<u>a</u>), and as the inactive form (GP<u>b</u>). It is interconverted by GPK and PP1G.

The presence of insulin promotes activation of phosphoprotein phosphatases which cleave enzyme phosphate groups, thereby activating GS and deactivating GP. Conversely, α- or ß-agonists activate cAMP- and Ca^{2+}-dependent protein kinases which increase the phosphate content and deactivate GS while activating GP [28-32]. This coordinated enzyme system is therefore exquisitely sensitive to the circulating hormonal milieu, and becomes disrupted in the diabetic state. Hypoinsulinemia leads to a reduced glycogen synthesis rate by promoting low GS activity, and is accompanied by an increased sensitivity of GP to catecholamine activation [4,5,33,34]. It is therefore somewhat paradoxical that the heart tends to store more glycogen than normal in the diabetic state. Treatment of diabetic animals with insulin normalizes the glycogen content and enzyme activities [4,19]. In the following two sections, the regulation of myocardial glycogen synthase and phosphorylase will be considered independently, along with the defects in each enzyme system associated with the diabetic state.

Glycogen synthase

GS occurs in two forms; the phosphorylated form is inactive by itself but is stimulated by glucose 6-phosphate (G6P) and is therefore called the *dependent-form* (GS<u>D</u>). Enzymatically-catalyzed activation of GS by the removal of covalently-bound phosphates yields the active form of GS which does not require G6P and is thus know as the *independent-form* (GS<u>I</u>). Rabbit skeletal muscle GS contains nine serine phosphorylation sites per subunit, and although the exact pattern of phosphate binding determines activity, the affinity for G6P is roughly inversely correlated with phosphate content [28,30,35-38]. Experimentally GS activity is determined by measuring the ability of tissue homogenate to promote incorporation of ^{14}C-UDPG into glycogen at both low and high concentrations of G6P. At low G6P levels the activity is reported as GS<u>I</u>, the active form, independent of G6P and at high G6P the activity represents the sum of GS<u>I</u> and GS<u>D</u>, or total activity. The ratio of the two measurements reflects the activation state of the enzyme, which is severely depressed in the diabetic heart [4,5,6,17,39,40].

GS<u>D</u> is activated predominantly by the glycogen-associated protein phosphatase-1 (PP1G) [27-30,37,38]. The activity of PP1G is directly regulated in response to both insulin and epinephrine [6,29-31,38,41], and is altered in diabetes. Figure 8.2 shows an outline of the covalent and allosteric regulation of glycogen synthase in response to insulin and epinephrine. PP1G is composed of a catalytic subunit (C) and a regulatory subunit (G) which is responsible for binding of the enzyme to glycogen. The G subunit can be phosphorylated at two serine sites, one of which stimulates (site 1), and one of which inactivates the enzyme (site 2). When G contains a single phosphate at site 1, association between C and G is promoted, and PP1G catalytic activity is expressed. Phosphorylation of site 2 always promotes subunit dissociation and enzyme inactivation. Site 1 is phosphorylated by an insulin-stimulated protein kinase, which then causes activation of PP1G enzyme activity and leads to GS$\underline{D}$ to GS$\underline{I}$ conversion and inactivation of glycogen phosphorylase.

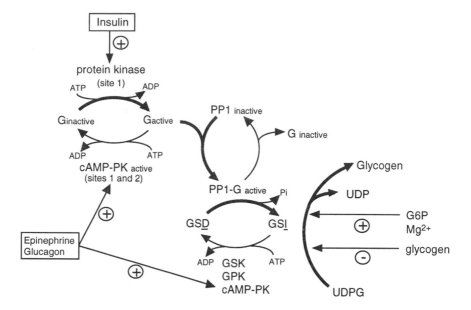

Figure 8.2: The regulation of glycogen synthase. Abbreviations are the same as in Fig.8.1, with the following additions: cAMP-dependent protein kinase (cAMP-PK); glycogen-binding regulatory subunit of PP1G (G). The pathway stimulated by insulin is shown in heavy lines. Insulin activates a protein kinase which phosphorylates site one on G, promoting association of PP1 and G. PP1G is then able to cleave phosphate from GS$\underline{D}$, forming GS$\underline{I}$. The activation of cAMP-PK leads to phosphorylation of site 2 of G, which causes dissociation of the two subunits, and deactivation of PP1-G.

In response to epinephrine, cAMP-dependent protein kinase (cAMP-PK) phosphorylates both sites (1 and 2) leading to inactivation of the C subunit [37], which is then unable to dephosphorylate GS$\underline{D}$. The phosphate on site 2 is the more labile of the two sites to protein phosphatase 2A, and therefore the G subunit loses this phosphate immediately upon withdrawal of epinephrine. It retains the phosphate at site 1 for a longer period of time, however, which causes reassociation and activation of PP1G [30]. This simple regulation of a protein phosphatase leads to high GS$\underline{I}$ and low GP$\underline{a}$ activity when insulin is present, and low GS$\underline{I}$ and high GP$\underline{a}$ activity as long as epinephrine is present. It also allows for immediate activation of GS$\underline{I}$ following the removal of epinephrine. This may be the mechanism which leads to the observed fast resynthesis of glycogen in the heart [30,42,43] (see below).

The serines on GS that are dephosphorylated by PP1G in response to insulin (C30, C34 and C38) are rephosphorylated by glycogen synthase kinase-3 [30]. GSI is the substrate for at least 4 other protein kinases: cAMP-dependent protein kinase (cAMP-PK), glycogen phosphorylase kinase, glycogen synthase kinase-4, and glycogen synthase kinase-5. Epinephrine or other ß-agonist binding causes activation of the enzyme AMP cyclase, and the resultant cAMP binds the two regulatory subunits of cAMP-PK, causing dissociation and subsequent activation of the cAMP-PK catalytic subunit. Cyclic-AMP-dependent protein kinase phosphorylates and activates glycogen phosphorylase kinase, which in turn activates glycogen phosphorylase and inactivates glycogen synthase [15, 41]. GSI is therefore inactivated in response to the counter-regulatory hormones epinephrine, glucagon or α-adrenergic agonists by the incorporation of about 2 phosphates per monomer [29-32].

Glucose-6-phosphate is the major allosteric promoter of GS activity. When bound to its regulatory site on the enzyme, it raises the V_{max} of the phosphorylated forms of the enzyme, and can therefore promote glycogen synthesis even in the absence of insulin. In addition, activation of GSD to GSI by PP1G is promoted by G6P binding to the substrate protein [44]. Muscle GSI is also activated by Mg^{2+}, and can be allosterically inhibited by ATP, inorganic phosphate (P_i), uridine triphosphate (UTP) and uridine diphosphate (UDP) [36, 45-46]. There is also evidence that covalent activation of cardiac synthase is stimulated following reduction of its product glycogen, such as occurs after anoxia, ischemia, or heavy exercise. Glycogen itself may be an inhibitor of PP1G activity [47].

In light of the normal response of heart to insulin which results in activation of GS and accumulation of glycogen, it is not surprising that glycogen metabolism should be reduced in the hypoinsulinemic diabetic state. The maximal net rate of glycogen synthesis in the hearts of 3-day alloxan diabetic animals infused with 1 U/min insulin, was measured by ^{13}C NMR during an infusion of [1-^{13}C]glucose, and is only about half that of control,

171

0.18 μmol/min g wet wt vs. 0.32 μmol/min g wet wt [4-6, 40]. This reduction in the maximal rate of glycogen synthesis is the result of a reduced basal GSI enzyme activity and a defective activation in response to insulin of both GS and glycogen synthase phosphatase (PP1G). In the normal animals, GSI activity increased from 0.19 to 0.33 μmol/min g wet wt in response to insulin. In the diabetics, GSI increased from 0.04 to only 0.1 μmol/min g wet wt when insulin was infused. The total activity GSD was not affected (0.77 μmol/min g wet wt in control vs 0.63 μmol/min g wet wt in diabetics) [6]. This defect can be appreciated more clearly with reference to the kinetic parameters of the enzyme measured in tissue homogenates. The V_{max} of GSI is reduced from 0.88 to 0.44 μmol/min g wet wt by three days of alloxan diabetes, and K_M (UDPG) is increased from 0.28 mM to 1.32 mM. The alteration becomes even more apparent after 60 min of glucose and insulin infusion, when the K_M for the substrate UDPG is decreased in controls to 0.082 mM, but only to 0.63 mM in diabetics [6]. Interestingly, although the rate of glycogen synthesis is drastically reduced from normal by diabetes (0.18 μmol/min g wet wt), it is considerably higher than the activity of GSI measured in homogenates of diabetic hearts (0.10 μmol/min g wet wt). This may be partially due to the elevated levels of G6P (0.31 vs. 0.11 μmol/g wet wt in controls) [6].

The changes in GS appear to be a direct effect of insulin withdrawal rather than an indirect consequence of the particular diabetic model, and are manifested in intact animals, perfused hearts from diabetic animals, and cardiomyocytes cultured in the absence of insulin. GSI is reduced relative to controls in hearts from both 3-day alloxan diabetic rats (from 28% to 10%) and BB/W spontaneously diabetic rats from which insulin had been withdrawn for 2 days (from 30% to 17%) [4,5]. In perfused hearts from normal rats, 10^{-8} M insulin stimulated GSI activity two-fold at 5 min, but insulin had no effect on synthase from either alloxan- or spontaneously diabetic rats [4,5].

Insulin and insulin-like growth factor-1 (IGF-1) have both been found to stimulate glycogen synthase activity in isolated cardiomyocytes in a time- and dose-dependent manner, and this effect is dampened by the presence of 0.1 mM palmitate. If cells from either normal or diabetic hearts were incubated for up to 48

172

hours in medium that contained no insulin or growth hormone, the ability of insulin or IGF-1 to stimulate glycogen synthase was subsequently lost, and glycogen synthase phosphatase activity was severely depressed. Therefore, insulin-deficient cell culture medium mimics the effect of insulin-withdrawal *in vivo* [48].

There is ample evidence that a duration of hypoinsulinemia results in low GSI activity, and a reduced GS activation as an acute response to insulin [4-6,13,40]. Both of these parameters are normalized after several hours of exposure to insulin, however, and this appears to be largely an effect on glycogen synthase phosphatase activity [4]. Glycogen synthase phosphatase activity is reduced in the diabetic heart, and is unaffected by short term insulin treatment [4-6,13,42]. When insulin is injected into diabetic animals 1-6 hours before heart perfusion, the synthase phosphatase activity is restored from 4 to 8 nmol/min g wet wt. Insulin is then able to activate GSI by more than 2-fold in the perfused heart [4,38]. If cycloheximide is injected into diabetic animals along with insulin, synthase phosphatase activity remains low, and the insulin-dependent GSD to I conversion is abolished. This demonstrates that the chronic action of insulin is dependent on protein synthesis [4]. Insulin therefore has a two-fold effect on glycogen metabolism; on the one hand it stimulates the phosphatase-catalyzed conversion of GSD to the active GSI in an acute time frame, and on the other hand it maintains the activity of the phosphatase molecule over a longer time frame so that acute activation can take place [4,38].

An interesting defect occurs in diabetic animals following exercise [14,15] or short periods of global hypoxia [42,54]. In normal animals, glycogen is broken down during these stresses, and is then rapidly repleted during recovery. This results in "supercompensation" to levels much higher than basal [15]. In ^{13}C NMR experiments done *in vivo* in rat heart, the rate of glycogen synthesis measured in the hour following three 90 sec periods of global hypoxia (0.5 μmol/min g wet wt) was 2-fold faster than the rate seen with maximal insulin. The increased rate of synthesis is the result of an activation of GSI to >90% of the total enzyme, and this activation is not dependent on infused insulin [42]. The activation seen both after exercise and hypoxia is severely depressed in diabetic animals, and results in negligible glycogen synthesis (0.03 μmol/min g wet wt following hypoxia) [15, 42]. GSI activity and glycogen synthesis are only partially restored with acute infusion of insulin (synthesis = 0.28 μmol glycogen/min g wet wt) [42]; however, treatment of the diabetic animals with insulin before exhaustive exercise normalizes the resultant glycogen supercompensation [15].

This lack of activation following hypoxia or exercise may be similar in origin to the altered response of GSI activity to epinephrine in diabetes. Rao *et al.* [49] noted that GSI was reduced from 27 to 18% during exposure of control perfused hearts to epinephrine, but was not changed from its basal level of 6% in the diabetic hearts. Similarly, GSI in normal isolated cardiomyocytes is deactivated from 35 to 25%, but is not altered by epinephrine in cells from diabetic animals [34, 50]. As noted above, rabbit skeletal muscle GS is phosphorylated and deactivated by exposure to epinephrine *in vivo*, then rapidly activated immediately upon epinephrine withdrawal. If a similar mechanism operates in heart, it may be disrupted in the hypoinsulinemic state.

Since glycogen synthase activity is so clearly diminished in diabetes, what does account for the increased myocardial glycogen stores seen in diabetes? In the healthy animal, the insulin released following a meal promotes glucose uptake and phosphorylation, glycolysis, and glycogen synthase activation, leading to glycogen storage in the heart. A second potent mechanism is also likely to be important in the normal heart, and may be effective in stimulating glycogen storage in diabetic heart. Glycogen synthesis is stimulated both *in vivo* and in perfused heart by the presence of high blood levels of free fatty acids, acetate, ketone bodies, lactate or pyruvate [38,51-53]. In the *in vivo* dog heart when maximal insulin was present, glycogen synthesis was stimulated more than five-fold by 10 mM lactate in the bloodstream [52]. In perfused hearts, 10 mM acetate or pyruvate increased glycogen accumulation from 2.2 to 14 μmol/g dry wt/hour if insulin was absent, or from 46 to 95 μmol/g dry wt/hour in its presence [38]. Therefore, the effect of non-glucose oxidizeable substrates can be much more important than insulin alone for promoting glycogen storage in the normal heart. The phenomenon appears to be an extension of the Randle free fatty acid cycle: the non-glucose substrate is oxidized preferentially in the mitochondria and results in inhibition of glycolysis at pyruvate dehydrogenase through elevated mitochondrial NADH and acetyl-CoA, and at phosphofructokinase (PFK) through elevated citrate and reduced fructose 2,6-phosphate [53,54]. Inhibition of glycolysis relative to glucose transport results in highly elevated G6P, which then stimulates GSD activity, inhibits GPa, and results in glycogen formation. G6P concentration is 0.223 μmol/gram in rat heart perfused with 11 mM glucose and 10 mM lactate, as opposed to 0.060 μmol/gram with glucose alone, or 0.147 μmol/gram with glucose and 7 μM insulin [53].

There is evidence that a differential between glucose phosphorylation and glycolysis exists in diabetic heart, leading to elevated G6P which could then promote glycogen storage. The plasma levels of substrates other than glucose, such as free fatty acids, triacylglycerols, and ketone bodies (ß-hydroxybutyrate and acetoacetate) are elevated [17]. The ability to oxidize glucose is severely reduced from 1.45 to 0.4 nmol/min mg protein in isolated cardiomyocytes from diabetic animals, although palmitate oxidation is unaltered, and ß-hydroxybutyrate oxidation is only slightly reduced [17, 19]. G6P is elevated in the rat heart at 12 weeks of experimental diabetes (703 nmol/g wet wt in diabetics vs. 351 in controls). Fructose-6-phosphate (23 nmol/g wet wt in diabetics vs. 10 in controls) and citrate (0.65 nmol/g wet wt in diabetics vs. 0.42 in control) are also high, whereas fructose-1,6-bisphosphate is reduced at all times, indicating that the major rate-limiting step is at PFK [17]. This is in spite of the fact that the activity of PFK measured in tissue homogenates is not reduced by diabetes [19].

This finding of elevated G6P is not universal in studies of diabetic heart, but it is usually in perfused heart that G6P appears to be low, and this is probably caused by perfusion with buffers that do not mimic the substrate and hormonal milieu found *in vivo* [7, 55, 56]. Myocardial G6P does appear to be elevated over control in many studies of experimental diabetes where hearts were freeze-clamped directly from the animal [6, 17, 39]. This high G6P may therefore result in persistent stimulation of GSD and elevated rates of myocardial glycogen storage over time, even though the rate of glycogen synthesis measured in acute experiments is reduced from normal.

175

Glycogen phosphorylase

Glycogen phosphorylase cleaves glycogen by addition of P_i to the outermost glucosyl moiety to produce G1P. Glycogen phosphorylase b (GPb) is inactive without its primary allosteric activator, AMP. It is converted to the active AMP-independent phosphorylated form (glycogen phosphorylase a, GPa) by the calcium-dependent glycogen phosphorylase kinase (GPK), which is in turn also activated by cAMP-PK [28, 33, 57]. GPa and GPb are usually measured in the non-physiological direction in tissue homogenates by ^{14}C-G1P incorporation into glycogen in the absence and presence of AMP, respectively.

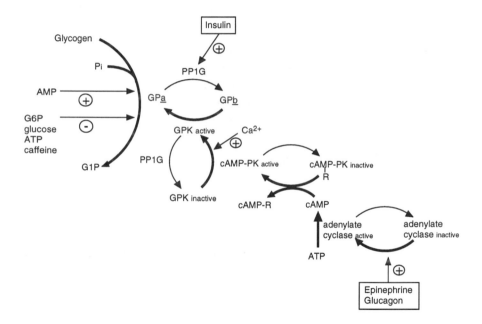

Figure 8.3: The regulation of glycogen phosphorylase. Abbreviations are the same as in Figs. 8.1 and 8.2, with the addition of the cAMP-bind regulatory subunit of cAMP-PK (cAMP-R). Adenylate cyclase is activated by epinephrine or glucagon, and the cAMP binds and releases cAMP-R from cAMP-PK, resulting in activation. cAMP-PK phosphorylates and activates GPK, which then activates GPb to GPa.

As in the glycogen synthase system, the regulatory kinases are directly activated by receptor binding of hormones such as epinephrine and glucagon (Figure 8.3). Activation of GPb to GPa by glucagon exposure (a ß-agonist) is immediate, followed by a slow return to basal activity (about 30 min *in vivo*), and glycogen breakdown follows a similar time course [58]. Interestingly, the activity of GP$\underline{a}$ measured in tissue homogenates is 5-6 times higher than the measured rate of glycogen breakdown [58]. Glycogen degradation also occurs during anoxia and ischemia. The rate is faster than can be accounted for by conversion of GP$\underline{b}$ to GP$\underline{a}$, and the elevated concentrations of the substrate P_i and primary activator AMP that result from ATP breakdown probably both stimulate GP$\underline{b}$ activity. Under other conditions, GP$\underline{a}$ activity can be inhibited by a battery of allosteric effectors including glucose, G6P and other phosphorylated sugars, ATP, and caffeine [59,60].

The behavior of GP in diabetic heart has been studied as glycogen breakdown in the intact animal, perfused heart, and cardiomyocyte, as enzyme activity in tissue homogenates, and in the purified enzyme. A variety of alterations have been found, but it is unclear which are most important for the heart metabolism of glycogen *in vivo*. Our discussion will begin with the original observation that cardiac glycogen concentration is increased during diabetes. The defects seen in the glycogen synthetic system of diabetic heart would apparently lead to a smaller pool of stored glycogen than normal, but only if the glycogen phosphorylase system is unaffected. If glycogen mobilization is also inhibited, it could eventually result in the observed increased glycogen. At first glance, this does not appear to be the case, since in normal heart insulin has no effect on glycogen phosphorylase activity or its activity ratio, GP$\underline{a}$/GP$\underline{b}$ [4-6]. GP$\underline{b}$ in either perfused hearts from diabetic animals or in isolated cardiomyocytes appears to have a near normal or slightly elevated basal activity of about 27 to 35 µmol/min/g wet wt and the activity of the activated form, GP$\underline{a}$ is also normal or elevated, equal to between 5% and 20% of the total GP$\underline{b}$ activity [5,6,33,49]. Hearts freeze-clamped without perfusion from diabetic animals will sometimes exhibit elevated GP$\underline{a}$ activity [64], but after a long period of anesthesia *in vivo*, the enzyme is similar to values from comparably-treated control animals [6]. Neither insulin nor diabetes have an effect on cAMP concentration or on the total or active cAMP-PK activity [4].

Although basal GP and cAMP-PK activity are unaltered by diabetes, exposure of the diabetic animal, perfused heart, or isolated cardiomyocytes to a ß-agonist appears to result in a hyper-stimulation of GP$\underline{a}$ activity and glycogen mobilization [5,33,34]. The mechanism for this is not readily apparent. When epinephrine is introduced to perfused hearts, those from BB/W spontaneously diabetic rats have a higher GP$\underline{a}$ activity (11.6 µmol/g wet wt min) than control (7.5 µmol/g wet. min) [5]. In other experiments, however, isoproterenol treatment of perfused hearts resulted in a similar increase in GP$\underline{a}$ activity to 60-70% of total GP in both 4 day alloxan-diabetic and control hearts, but the glycogen concentration fell much more quickly in the diabetic hearts than in controls [33]. This increased ability for a given amount of enzyme activity to break down glycogen may partially be a function of the fact that the diabetic hearts have much more glycogen to begin with, so the total exposed surface area of the particles is much larger (which is equal to the available substrate for GP).

Even though the activation of glycogen phosphorylase after ß-agonist exposure was similar to controls or elevated, the cAMP concentration was either constant (with epinephrine) or increased only 2-fold (with isoproterenol) in diabetic heart as opposed to the 4-fold seen in controls [5,33]. The activated cAMP-PK was 40% of total in diabetics compared to 60% in controls, and correlation analysis shows that the cAMP-PK activation ratio bears the same linear relationship to cAMP in normal and diabetic heart [33]. Similar observations have been made in long-term alloxan or streptozotocin diabetic rats, where the cAMP response to isoproterenol was normal in perfused hearts from diabetics, but the GP$\underline{a}$ was activated to 50% in diabetics as opposed to only 25% in controls [49].

This hypersensitivity of phosphorylase activation and/or glycogen breakdown in the presence of epinephrine has been studied extensively in primary cultures of cardiomyocytes from diabetic animals by Miller and his colleagues. They determined that the rate of synthesis of phosphorylase protein is similar in normal and diabetic cardiomyocytes, although it is drastically reduced by diabetes in hepatocytes [62]. Glycogen phosphorylase is activated by epinephrine from the same basal level of 11% to 32% in diabetic cardiomyocytes as opposed to 25% in normal cells, and the half-maximal dose of epinephrine is reduced from a control value of 1×10^{-6} M to 5×10^{-7} M in diabetics. The effects of epinephrine on phosphorylase appear to be a pure ß-agonist effect, since no effect is elicited by phenylephrine, an α_1-agonist, and the epinephrine effect can be blocked by 10 µM propranolol (a ß$_1$/ß$_2$ antagonist) but not by prazosin, a selective α_1-receptor antagonist [50]. Therefore activation of glycogen phosphorylase seems to be selectively more responsive to ß-adrenergic stimulation in hearts from diabetic than from normal animals. This appears to be a property of the glycogen phosphorylase molecule itself, not of cAMP production or protein kinase activation, and indicates that the diabetic state may result in a phosphorylase protein that is a better substrate for its activating protein kinase.

The behavior of ß-adrenergic receptors to epinephrine have also been studied in diabetic cardiomyocytes [63-66]. Diabetic heart has a smaller inotropic response to catecholamines, and this has been ascribed to a reduced cell surface concentration of ß-receptors [63,64]. Beta-receptors exist in an intracellular pool and are recruited to the cell surface where they become active. In turn, the surface receptor concentration is reduced in response to catecholamine binding [65]. The total cellular receptor concentration and equilibrium dissociation constant are similar for diabetics and controls [66]; however, the active receptor concentration found on the cell surface is reduced by diabetes from 155 to 92 fmol/10^6 cells [58]. Insulin treatment for 48 hours *in vivo*, (but not *in vitro*) normalized the number of surface receptors [62]. Therefore, there appears to be no diabetes-associated defect in ß-adrenergic receptor synthesis, but recruitment from the intracellular storage pool to the active membrane-bound population is attenuated [66]. These data fail to explain the hypersensitivity of glycogen phosphorylase to activation by ß-agonists.

Berndt and Rosen [67-69] purified the glycogen phosphorylase protein from normal and diabetic hearts and found kinetic alterations due to the diabetic state. Hearts from both normal and diabetic rats contained two isozymes of glycogen phosphorylase (isozymes I and II). Both of these proteins are activated through the action of glycogen phosphorylase kinase by the incorporation of one mole phosphate per mole subunit enzyme. The ratio of the isozymes (I / II $\approx$ 4) is not affected by diabetes. Despite the fact that basal phosphorylase activity is unaltered by diabetes, the yield of total purified protein was reduced to 50% of controls, possibly indicating an increased sensitivity to proteinases during purification. Defects were found in both the allosteric regulation of the diabetic protein and in its kinetic activity. GP-Ia from diabetic animals was shown to have a lower affinity for its substrates glycogen and P_i than the enzyme from normal animals. Both diabetic isozymes I and II were more slowly phosphorylated (activated) by rabbit skeletal muscle phosphorylase kinase, but both were dephosphorylated at the same rate as control enzyme by protein phosphatase. A unique property of the diabetic isozymes is that although they are dephosphorylated at the same rates as the proteins from normal animals, they are deactivated twice as fast; that is, covalently attached phosphate content and the enzyme activity are no longer linearly related, and the diabetic enzyme has a lower activity at a given phosphate concentration [69]. Therefore, the diabetic defect in the isolated glycogen phosphorylase protein appears as a reduction in the affinity for the substrate, in a lower rate of activation by skeletal muscle glycogen phosphorylase kinase, and in an increase in the rate of deactivation. If expressed *in vivo*, these alterations in GP would result in reduced glycogen turnover and a higher net glycogen synthetic rate at a given glycogen synthase activity. The kinetic properties of the isolated enzyme therefore may partially explain the increased glycogen concentration found in the diabetic heart.

Role of increased glycogen

Since increased glycogen in the face of sluggish and unresponsive glycogen metabolism seems to be a universal finding in the diabetic heart, one wonders if this potential substrate pool serves a protective role during ischemia or anoxia. Glycogen appears to be protective during short periods of anoxia in the normal heart [13], and would logically also serve to maintain function in the diabetic heart during increased stress.

When unstressed, diabetic perfused hearts oxidize much less total glucose than controls (718 vs. 403 nmol/min g wet wt). At low work loads, the diabetic heart does mobilize a larger amount of glycogen than controls (542 vs. 455 nmol/min g wet wt) and of this an equal amount is oxidized (379 vs. 341 nmol/min g wet wt) [1]. In the face of low-flow ischemia with norepinephrine, the perfused diabetic heart exhibits a faster decline in oxygen consumption, peak systolic pressure, and cardiac output, although the post-ischemic glycogen concentration is similar to normals [70]. Function and ultrastructural damage incurred during reflow after 30 min of regional ischemia is worse in the diabetic myocardium, and unlike control hearts, no resynthesis of glycogen is seen [71]. Pre-treatment of the diabetic hearts with insulin before low-flow ischemia results in increased function, phosphocreatine and ATP levels, but there was no protective effect of insulin when it was included only during the reduced flow period [72]. Therefore, the excess glycogen pool found in diabetic hearts and the increased ability to mobilize it, do not appear to protect the heart in the face of ischemia.

Summary

The diabetic cardiac myopathy is associated with altered glycogen metabolism. Glycogen stores are dramatically increased, and the concentration correlates with duration and severity of disease. Paradoxically, the rates of glycogen synthesis measured in intact animals and in perfused hearts are very low, caused both by reduced basal glycogen synthase activity and a resistance to enzyme activation in response to insulin. Diabetic heart exhibits an increased sensitivity to epinephrine despite a lower concentration of ß-receptors on the cell surface. This results in an enhanced ability of epinephrine to activate glycogen phosphorylase and cause glycogen mobilization. The diabetic defects in glycogen metabolism can be reversed in a few hours by treatment with insulin *in vivo*.

References

1. Rosen T, Windeck P, Zimmer H-G, Frenzel H, Burring KF and Reinauer H. Myocardial performance and metabolism in non-ketotic diabetic rat hearts: myocardial function and metabolism *in vivo* and in the isolated perfused heart under the influence of insulin and octanoate. *Basic Res. Cardiol.* **81**: 620-635, 1986.

2. Kerbey AL, Radcliffe PM and Randle PJ. Diabetes and the control of pyruvate dehydrogenase in rat heart mitochondria by concentration ratios of adenosine triphosphate/adenosine diphosphate, or reduced/oxidized nicotinamide adenine dinucleotide and of acetyl CoA/CoA. *Biochem. J.* **164**: 509-519, 1977.

3. Kobayashi K and Neely JR. Effects of increased cardiac work on pyruvate dehydrogenase activity in hearts from diabetic animals. *J. Mol. Cell. Cardiol.* **15**: 347-57, 1983.

4. Miller TB. A dual role for insulin in the regulation of cardiac glycogen synthase. *J. Biol. Chem.* **253**. 5389-5394, 1978.

5. Miller TB. Altered regulation of cardiac glycogen metabolism in spontaneously diabetic rats. *Am J. Physiol.* **245**: E379-E383, 1983.

6. Laughlin MR, Petit WA, Shulman RG and Barrett EJ. Measurement of myocardial glycogen synthesis in diabetic and fasted rats. *Am. J. Physiol.* **258**: E184-E190, 1990.

7. Opie LH, Mansford KRL and Owen P. Effects of increased heart work on glycolysis and adenine nucleotides in the perfused heart of normal and diabetic rats. *Biochem. J.* **124**: 475-490, 1971.

8. Denton RM and Randle PJ. Concentration of glycerides and phospholipids in rat heart and gastrocnemus muscle. Effects of alloxan-diabetes and perfusion. *Biochem. J.* **194**: 416-422, 1967.

9. Garland PB and Randle PJ. Regulation of glucose uptake by muscle. X. Effect of alloxan diabetes, starvation. *Biochem. J.* **93**: 678-687, 1964.

10. Garland PB, Newsholme EA and Randle PJ. Citrate as an intermediary in inhibition of PFK in rat heart and muscle by free fatty acids, ketone bodies, pyruvate, diabetes and starvation. *Nature* **200**: 169-70, 1963.

11. Neely JR and Morgan HE. Relationship between carbohydrate and lipid metabolism and the energy balance of heart muscle. *Ann. Rev. Physiol.* **36**: 413-459, 1974.

12. Regen DM, Davis WW, Morgan HE and Park CR. The regulation of hexokinase and phosphofructokinase acitivity in heart muscle. *J. Biol. Chem.* **241**: 632-649, 1964.

13. Scheuer J and Stezoski SW. Protective role of increased myocardial glycogen stores in cardiac anoxia in the rat. *Circ. Res.* **27**: 835-849, 1970.

14. Segel LH and Mason, DT. Effects of exercise and conditioning on rat heart glycogen and glycogen synthase. *J. Appl. Physiol.* **44**: 183-190, 1978.

15. Conlee RK and Tipton CM. Cardiac glycogen repletion after exercise: influence of synthase and glucose-6-phosphate. *J. Appl. Physiol.* **42**: 240-44, 1977.

16. Poland JL and Blount DH. Glycogen depletion in rat ventricles during graded exercise. *Proc. Soc. Exptl. Biol. Med.* **121**: 560-562, 1966.

17. Chen V, Ianuzzo CD, Fong BC and Spitzer JJ. The effects of acute and chronic diabetes on myocardial metabolism in rats. *Diabetes* **33**: 1078-84, 1984.

18. Hamilton N, Noble EG and Ianuzzo CD. Glycogen repletion in different skeletal muscles from diabetic rats. *Am. J. Physiol.* **247**: E740-E746, 1984.

19. Chen V, and Ianuzzo CD. Dosage effect of streptozotocin on rat tissue enzyme activities and glyocgen concentration. *Can. J. Physiol. Pharmacol.* **60**: 1251-1256, 1982.

20. Ianuzzo CD, Noble EG, Hamilton N and Dabrowski B. Effects of streptozotocin diabetes, insulin treatment, and training on the diaphragm. *J. Appl. Physiol.* **52**: 1471-1475, 1982.

21. Bhimji S, Godin DV and McNeill JH. Myocardial ultrastructural changes in alloxan-induced diabetes in rabbits. *Acta Anat.* **125**: 195-200, 1986.

22. Jackson CV, McGrath GM, Tahiliani AG, Vadlamudi RVSV and McNeill GH. A functional and ultrastructural analysis of experimental diabetic rat myocardium. *Diabetes* **34**: 876-883, 1985.

23. Hsiao YC, Suzuki K, Abe H and Toyota T. Ultrastructural alterations in cardiac muscle of diabetic BB Wistar Rats. *Virchows Archiv A*, **411**: 45-52, 1987.

24. Xi Z, Zhou X, Zhong X, Zhong C and Yu Y. Streptozotocin induced cardiomyopathy in diabetic rats. *Chinese Medical J.* **106**: 463-466, 1993.

25. Drochmans P. Morphologie du glycogene. *J. Ultrastructure Res.* **6**. 141-163, 1962.

26. Wanson JJ and Drochmans P. Rabbit skeletal muscle glycogen. A morphological and biochemical study of glycogen ß-particles. *J. Cell Biol.* **38**: 130-150, 1968.

27. Villar-Pallasi C and Larner J. Glycogen metabolism and glycolytic enzymes. *Ann. Rev. Biochem.* **39**: 639-672, 1970.

28. Cohen P. The role of protein phosphorylation in the hormonal control of enzyme activity. *Eur. J. Biochem.* **151**: 439-448, 1985.

29. Ramachandran C, Angelos KL and Walsh DA. Hormonal regulation of the phosphorylation of glycogen synthase in perfused rat heart: effects of insulin, catecholamines, and glucagon. *J. Biol. Chem.* **258**: 13377-13383, 1983.

30. Dent P, Lavoinne A, Nakielny S, Caudwell FB, Watt P and Cohen P. The molecular mechanism by which insulin stimulates glycogen synthesis in mammalian skeletal muscle. *Nature* **348**: 302-308, 1990.

31. Blackmore PJ, Strickland G, Bocckino SB and Exton JH. Mechanism of hepatic glycogen synthase inactivation induced by Ca^{2+}-mobilizing hormones. *Biochem. J.* **237**: 235-242, 1986.

32. Parker PJ, Embi N, Caudwell FB and Cohen P. Glycogen synthase from rabbit skeletal muscle. *Eur. J. Biochem.* **124**: 47-55, 1982.

33. Ingebretsen C, Peralta M, Monsher M, Wagner LK and Ingebretsen CG. Diabetes alters the myocardial cAMP-protein kinase cascade system. *Am. J. Physiol.* **240**: H375-H382, 1981.

34. Wolleben CD, Jaspers SR and Miller TB. Use of adult rat cardiomyocytes to study cardiac glycogen metabolism. *Am. J. Physiol.* **252**: E6743-E678, 1987.

35. Nuttall FQ and Gannon MC. An improved assay for hepatic glycogen synthase in liver extracts with emphasis on synthase R *Anal. Biochem.* **178**: 311-319, 1989.

36. Roach PJ, Takeda Y and Larner J. Rabbit skeletal muscle glycogen synthase.I. Relationship between phosphorylation states and kinetic properties. *J. Biol. Chem.* **251**: 1913-1919, 1976.

37. Cohen P. The structure and regulation of protein phosphatases. *Ann. Rev. Biochem.* **58**: 453-508, 1989.

38. Nuttall FQ, Gannon MC, Corbett VA and Wheeler MP. Insulin stimulation of heart glycogen synthase D phosphatase (protein phosphatase). *J. Biol. Chem.* **251**: 6724-6729, 1976.

39. Das I. Studies on glycogen metabolism in normal and diabetic rat heart *in vivo*. *Can. J. Biochem.* **51**: 637-641, 1973.

40. Chain EB, Mansford KRL and Opie LH. Effects of insulin on the pattern of glucose metabolism in the perfused working and Langendorff heart of normal and insulin-deficient rats. *Biochem. J.* **115**: 537-546, 1969.

41. Embi N, Parker PJ and Cohen P. A reinvestigation of the phosphorylation of rabbit skeletal muscle glycogen synthase by cyclic-AMP-dependent protein kinase. *Eur. J. Biochem.* **115**: 405-413, 1980.

42. Laughlin MR, Morgan C and Barrett EJ. Hypoxemeic stimulation of heart glyocgen synthase and synthesis: effects of insulin and diabetes mellitus. *Diabetes* **40**: 385-90, 1991.

43. Laughlin MR, Taylor JF, Chesnick AS and Balaban RS. Regulation of glycogen metabolism in canine myocardium: effects of insulin and epinephrine *in vivo*. *Am. J. Physiol.* **262**: E875-E883, 1992.

44. Villar-Palasi C. Substrate specific activation by glucose-6-phosphate of the dephosphorylation of muscle glycogen synthase. *Biochim. Biophys. Acta* **1095**: 216-267, 1991.

45. Nakai C and Thomas JA. Effects of magnesium on the kinetic properties of bovine heart glycogen synthase D. *J. Biol. Chem.* **250**: 4081-4086, 1975.

46. Piras R, Rothman LB and Cabib E. Regulation of muscle glycogen synthetase by metabolites: differential effects on the I and D forms. *Biochemistry* **7**: 56-66, 1968.

47. Mellgren RL and Coulson M. Coordinated feedback regulation of muscle glycogen metabolism: inhibition of purified phosphorylase phosphatase by glycogen. *Biochem. Biophys. Res. Commun.* **114**: 148-154, 1983.

48. Jaspers SR, Garnache AK, and Miller TB. Factors affecting the activation of glycogen synthase in primary culture cardiomyocytes. *J. Mol. Cell. Cardiol.* **25**: 1171-1178, 1993.

49. Vadlamudi RVSV and McNeill JH. Effect of experimental diabetes on rat cardiac cAMP, phosphorylase and inotropy. *Am. J. Physiol.* **244**: H844-H851, 1983

50. Buczek-Thomas J, Jaspers SR and Miller TB. Adrenergic activation of glycogen phosphorylase in primary culture diabetic cardiomyocytes. *Am. J. Physiol.* **262**: H649-H653, 1992.

51. Nakao M, Matsubara T and Sakamoto N. Effects of diabetes on cardiac glycogen metabolism in rats. *Heart Vessels (Japan)* **8**: 171-5, 1993.

52. Laughlin MR, Taylor J, Chesnick AS and Balaban RS. Nonglucose substrates increase glycogen synthesis *in vivo* in dog heart. *Am. J. Physiol.* **267**: H217-H223, 1994.

53. Depre C, Veitch K and Hue L. Role of fructose-2,6-bisphosphate in the control of glycolysis. Stimulation of glycogen synthesis by lactate in the isolated working rat heart. *Acta Cardiol.* **48**: 147-164, 1993.

54. Randle PJ. Regulation of glycolysis and pyruvate oxidation in cardiac muscle. *Circ. Res.* **38**(suppl 1): I-8 - I-15, 1976.

55. Das I. Effects of heart work and insulin on glycogen metabolism in the perfused rat heart. *Am. J. Physiol.* **224**: 7-12, 1973.

56. Schaffer SW, Mozaffari MS, Cutcliff CR and Wilson GL. Postreceptor myocardial metabolic defect in a rat model of non-insulin-dependent diabetes mellitus. *Diabetes* **35**: 593-97, 1986.

57. Rasmussen H. The calcium messenger system. *N. Engl. J. Med.* **314**: 1094-1101 and 1164-1170, 1986.

58. Laughlin MR, Petit WA and Barrett EJ. The time course of myocardial glyocgenolysis stimulated by glucagon. *J. Mol. Cell. Cardiol.* **25**: 175-183, 1993.

59. Yamada T and Sugi H. ^{31}P-NMR study of the regulation of glycogenolysis in living skeletal muscle. *Biochim. Biophys. Acta* **931**: 170-174. 1987.

60. Griffiths JR. Non-covalent control of glycogenolysis in muscle. in *Short-term regulation of liver metabolism*, ed. Hue L and Van de Werve G. Elsevier/North-Holland Biomedical Press, 1981. pp.77-91.

61. Chaudhuri SN and Shipp JC. Cyclic AMP in hearts of alloxan-diabetic rats. *Recent Adv. Stud. Cardiac Struct. Metab.* **3**: 319-330, 1973.

62. Rulfs J, Jaspers SR, Garnache AK and Miller TB. Phosphorylase synthesis in diabetic hepatocytes and cardiomyocytes. *Am J. Physiol.* **257**: E74-E80, 1989.

63. Götzsche O. The adrenergic ß-receptor, adenylate cyclase system in heart and lymphocytes from streptozotocin-diabetic rats. *In vivo* and *in vitro* evidence for a desensitized myocardial ß-receptor. *Diabetes* **32**: 1110-1116, 1983.

64. Savareses JJ and Berkowitz BA. ß-Adrenergic receptor decrease in diabetic rat heart. *Life Sci.* **25**: 2075-2078, 1979.

65. Stiles GL, Caron MG and Lefkowitz RJ. ß-Adrenergic receptors: biochemical mechanism of physiological regulation. *Physiol. Rev.* **64**: 661-743, 1983.

66. Kashiwagi A, Nishio Y, Saeki Y, Kida Y, Kodama M and Shigeta Y. Plasma membrane-specific deficiency in cardiac ß-receptor in streptozocin-diabetic rats. *Am. J. Physiol.* **257**: E127-E132, 1989.

67. Berndt N and Rosen P. Isolation and partial characterization of two forms of rat heart glycogen phosphorylase. *Arch. Biochem. Biophys.* **228**: 143-154, 1984.

68. Berndt N, Neubauer HP and Rosen P. Rat heart glycogen phosphorylase-II is genetically distinct from phosphorylase-I. *Biochim. Biophys. Acta* **915**: 217-224, 1987.

69. Berndt N and Rosen R. Activation and inactivation of glycogen phosphorylase isoenzymes purified from the diabetic rat heart. *Eur. J. Biochem.* **21**: 355-360, 1989.

70. Lopashuk GD and Spafford MA. Acute insulin withdrawal contributes to ischemic heart failure in spontaneously diabetic BB wistar rats. *Can. J. Physiol. Pharmacol.* **68**: 462-466, 1990.

71. Bhimji S, Godin DV and McNeill JH. Coronary artery ligation and reperfusion in alloxan-diabetic rabbits: ultrastructural and haemodynamic changes. *Br. J. Exp. Path.* **67**: 851-863, 1986.

72. Ikema S, Higuchi M, Hirayama K and Sakanashi M. Improvement of hypoperfusion with norepinephrine injury by ex vivo insulin in isolated diabetic rat hearts. *Japan. J. Pharmacol.* **54**: 299-306, 1990.

CHAPTER 9

The Effect of Diabetes on Glucose Metabolism

John C. Chatham

Introduction

An association between diabetes and heart disease is not new; in the late 1800s heart failure was recognized as a frequent complication in diabetes mellitus [1]. It was also around this time that it was first suggested that heart disease in diabetic patients may be related to an abnormality in metabolism [2]. Studies from the early 1900s showed an increasing understanding of the effects of diabetes on the heart. Knowlton and Starling [3] noted that the inability of the diabetic heart to oxidize sugar was "the most prominent feature of the disorder". The availability of insulin enabled more detailed investigations to be carried out on the effects of diabetes on cardiac metabolism, and it was suggested by Cruickshank that the diabetic heart relied on oxidation of lipids due to impaired oxidation of carbohydrates [4]. These early studies provided the foundation for the multitude of investigations into the changes in cardiac metabolism wrought by diabetes mellitus that began in earnest with the studies by Morgan and colleagues [5-7] and Randle and co-workers [8-12] in the early 1960s and have continued to the present day.

The focus of this chapter is the effect of diabetes on glucose metabolism and it has been divided into separate sections on glucose transport and phosphorylation, glycolysis (i.e. metabolism from glucose 6-phosphate to pyruvate and lactate) and glucose oxidation. There is also a section devoted to the effects of diabetes on pyruvate dehydrogenase, since this enzyme complex plays a critical role in the regulation of glucose oxidation. The information presented in these sections is focused on studies of experimental models of diabetes; however, since we are ultimately interested in the effects of diabetes on the heart in humans, there will also be a summary of what is known about myocardial glucose utilization in diabetic patients.

__Glucose transport and phosphorylation__

Transport and phosphorylation of glucose are the essential first steps in the utilization of glucose, whether for oxidative metabolism, or for storage as glycogen. Decreased glucose uptake in diabetic hearts was observed as early as 1912 [3]; however, it was unknown whether this was due to alterations in transport and phosphorylation, or a decrease in oxidative metabolism. In an elegant series of studies, Morgan and colleagues in the early 1960s, investigated the regulation of glucose uptake in isolated perfused hearts from both normal and diabetic rats [5,6,13]. They separated glucose uptake into three steps -- 1) extracellular transfer of glucose from the capillary to the cell membrane; 2) transport of glucose across the cell membrane and 3) phosphorylation of glucose. The extracellular transfer of glucose was very rapid and was not a limiting step in glucose uptake. In the absence of insulin, transport of glucose appeared to be the limiting step for uptake; however, following the addition of insulin, phosphorylation was limiting for all glucose concentrations above 25mg/100ml (i.e., >1.4mM). In hearts from acutely diabetic animals (i.e., sacrificed 48 hours following 60mg/kg of alloxan monohydrate) a similar situation was observed with transport being the limiting step in the absence of insulin. Under all conditions, however, the actual rates of transport and phosphorylation were significantly depressed in diabetic hearts compared to controls. At low glucose concentrations (i.e., 2.8mM) without insulin, glucose transport and phosphorylation rates in diabetic hearts were approximately 60% of control values. While the addition of insulin increased these rates in both groups, the diabetic group was still only 70% of control values. Even under

190

conditions of maximal glucose uptake (i.e., high glucose, 22mM plus insulin), glucose transport and phosphorylation in diabetic hearts were still only 55-65% of control values. They concluded that the principal effects of diabetes was to decrease the apparent V_{max} for glucose transport by more than two fold and increase the K_m for glucose phosphorylation by more than 7 fold.

These studies were among the first detailed investigation of glucose utilization in diabetic hearts. Although the model that was used was an acute, very severe diabetes (animals died 3-4 days after treatment), the fundamental conclusions have been found to hold true in many experimental models of diabetes including spontaneously diabetic animals. That is, following diabetes myocardial glucose transport and phosphorylation are depressed compared to control. However, these studies did not determine whether changes in transport and phosphorylation are a result of decreased activity of the glucose transporters or hexokinase, an altered response of these proteins to glucose and/or insulin or a decrease in the concentration of these proteins in the tissue.

Glucose transporters

Glucose transport is mediated by a family of glucose transporter proteins (GLUT) two isoforms of which, GLUT1 and GLUT4, are expressed in muscle. GLUT1 is found in a wide range of tissues independent of whether glucose transport is regulated by insulin. In contrast GLUT4 is found primarily in insulin sensitive tissues, such as fat, skeletal and cardiac muscle. In cardiac muscle GLUT4 is the predominant isoform. Diabetes has consistently been shown to decrease the total GLUT4 protein levels [14-16], GLUT4 mRNA levels [17,18] , or both [19,20] in the heart.

In sarcolemmal vesicles isolated from hearts of normal and 4 week streptozotocin-diabetic rats Garvey et al. [20] were able to show that decreased rates of glucose transport in the diabetic group could be explained by a reduction in the number of GLUT4 transporters with normal activity. This decrease in GLUT4 protein corresponded to a decrease in GLUT4 mRNA suggesting that the impaired glucose transport in the heart following diabetes was due to pretranslational suppression of GLUT4 gene expression. Insulin treatment reversed these effects. In an acute diabetic model (72 hours after STZ treatment) a reduction in myocardial GLUT4 mRNA, but not protein content, was observed [18]; insulin treatment also reversed these effects. These two studies are consistent with the work of Kahn et al. [21], who reported that in skeletal muscle GLUT4 mRNA levels are decreased at both 7·and 14 days after induction of diabetes, but total GLUT4 protein is only decreased after 14 days of diabetes. Thus it appears that the decrease in myocardial glucose transport following diabetes is a result of a decrease in the synthesis of GLUT4 protein rather than an alteration in the function of the transporter or an increase in transporter degradation.

It is unclear whether the alterations in myocardial GLUT4 mRNA and protein levels of diabetic animals is due to a decrease in insulin or the result of an increase in serum glucose. Burcelin et al. found that while insulin treatment normalized GLUT4 mRNA levels, the hypoglycemic agent phlorizin (which blocks renal glucose reabsorption thus lowering serum glucose) did not. They concluded, therefore, that the regulation of GLUT4 synthesis was controlled by insulin [18]. In contrast, based on studies in skeletal muscle, Klip et al. [22] concluded that serum glucose levels regulates the biosynthesis of GLUT4. While these differences may be due to altered regulation in skeletal muscle versus cardiac muscle they may be also be due to the fact that Burcelin et al. [18] examined animals after only 72 hours following induction of diabetes. In the study by Klip and co-workers [22], treatment with phlorizin was started 5 days following streptozotocin treatment and continued for 3 days. This resulted in normal fasting glucose levels as well as normal GLUT4 (and GLUT1) transporter levels in the plasma membrane. It should be noted however, that phlorizin did not normalize the intracellular membrane pool of GLUT4.

Hexokinase activity

The reported effects of diabetes on myocardial hexokinase activity have been variable. England and Randle reported that net hexokinase activities in extracts from normal and alloxan diabetic rats were identical [23]. More recently Chen et al. [24] also observed that the activity of hexokinase was not altered in hearts from rats that had been diabetic for 48 hours, 4 or 12 weeks. In control, one month following STZ-induced diabetes in rats, Sochor et al. [25] reported a modest 20% decline in total hexokinase activity, resulting from a 60% decrease in type II hexokinase activity and 20% increase in hexokinase I. It is the presence of these different isoforms of hexokinase that may account for the contradictory reports on the effects of diabetes on hexokinase activity in the heart. In the rat heart the soluble fraction of hexokinase consists of principally of types I and II, with K_m values of 0.045mM and 0.25mM respectively [26]. In the study by England and Randle they reported the K_m in normal hearts to be 0.045mM, suggesting that they were preferentially measuring type I hexokinase. This could occur due to the relative instability of type II relative to type I [26]. It has been reported that in insulin sensitive tissues it is principally type II hexokinase that is effected by diabetes [27-29].

Katzen et al. [28], studied the multiple forms of hexokinase associated with both the soluble and subcellular particulate fractions in tissues of normal and diabetic rats. They reported that after 2-3 weeks of streptozotocin-induced diabetes, total soluble hexokinase was significantly less (40-50% less) than normal. This decrease in total activity was due entirely to a decline in the activity of type II hexokinase; diabetes had no effect on type I. Similar results were found after 5 weeks of diabetes. Within 3 days of diabetes, hexokinase activities were decreased in all the subcellular particulate fractions of the heart; no further changes were observed after 10 days of diabetes. As with the soluble fraction the decreased total activity was due to a loss of type II rather than type I hexokinase; however, the effects were even more pronounced. In contrast to the soluble fraction, where some type II activity persisted following diabetes, there was complete loss of particulate type II activity.

While the studies by Katzen clearly showed the effects of insulin deprivation on hexokinase activity, they did not determine whether this was due to an alteration in the regulation of hexokinase synthesis. More recently Burcelin et al. [18]. investigated the effects of short term diabetes on hexokinase activity and mRNA levels in the heart. Two to three days following STZ treatment hexokinase II activity was found to be decreased by approximately 25%; this corresponded to a similar decline in hexokinase II mRNA. The effect of diabetes was reversed by insulin treatment but not by phlorizin. If insulin treatment was stopped, hexokinase II mRNA rapidly (i.e., within 6 hours) fell to levels comparable with the untreated diabetic group. As with the studies by Katzen *et al.* [28] hexokinase I activity and mRNA levels were not affected by diabetes. These data suggest that it is the low levels of insulin rather than high levels of glucose that result in the decrease in hexokinase II expression and activity.

Glycolysis

The principal rate limiting reaction in glycolysis is the conversion of fructose 6-phosphate to fructose 1,6-diphosphate catalyzed by phosphofructokinase (PFK). In the early 1960s it was observed that in diabetic rats, there was an increase in myocardial glucose 6-phosphate and a decrease in fructose 1,6-diphosphate [30-33]. It was concluded that this was a due to decreased PFK activity. Subsequently, it was shown that similar changes were observed in hearts from normal rats perfused with fatty acids or ketone bodies [8]. It was proposed that both in hearts from diabetic animals and in hearts perfused with fatty acids (or ketone bodies) PFK activity was inhibited by an increase in citrate concentration. However, the reported effects of diabetes on measured PFK activity in the heart are somewhat variable. For example, Sochor *et al.* [25] reported a 20% decline in myocardial PFK activity in 3 week diabetic rats whereas Chen and co-workers [24,34] reported no change in activity even after 12 weeks of diabetes [24]. If the decreased activity in PFK is due to elevated levels of citrate, or some other intracellular effector, it is possible that this regulation could be lost in the preparation of tissue homogenates. Even though there was no difference in PFK activity Chen *et al.* [24] confirmed the earlier observations of increased glucose 6-phosphate and fructose 6-phosphate and decreased fructose 1,6-diphosphate. They also found an elevation in citrate concentration in myocytes from diabetic rats compared to non-diabetic controls. It is interesting to note that while the differences in sugar phosphates between the control and diabetic groups became greater with increasing duration of diabetes, the citrate levels were highest (250% of control) in the 48 hour diabetic group and lowest (150% of control) after 12 weeks of diabetes. This raises the possibility that elevations in citrate may be involved in

194

the short term regulation of PFK in the acute diabetic animal, but suggests that there may be an adaptive response that occurs as the duration of diabetes increases.

Measurements of the rate of glycolysis following diabetes arc variable, ranging from 23% to 97% of control [9,12,35-37]. For example, Randle and colleagues [9,12] showed that there was a marked decrease (30-50%) in the rate of myocardial glycolysis where --

glycolysis = (glucose uptake) - (intracellular glucose + change in glycogen)

In other words they defined the net glycolytic flux as the sum of the fluxes from pyruvate to lactate and pyruvate to acetyl-CoA. In control hearts, the formation of lactate and pyruvate represented about 30% of the total flux through glycolysis [9]. While glycolysis was depressed in the diabetic rats the rate of lactate and pyruvate efflux was unchanged and represented approximately 45% of the total glycolytic flux. Thus the difference between the total glycolytic flux and the lactate and pyruvate efflux in these studies reflects the rate of glucose oxidation; that is the decrease in total glycolytic flux in diabetic hearts was due principally to a decrease at the level of pyruvate oxidation rather than a decrease in flux through PFK. If glucose metabolism in diabetic hearts was principally limited by flux through PFK a decrease in lactate and pyruvate efflux would have been expected. This was similar to the study reported by Opie *et al.* [35] in the Langendorff perfused heart; they found that total glycolytic flux (i.e., pyruvate and lactate efflux plus $^{14}CO_2$ production) was decreased approximately 50% in hearts from diabetic animals, however, this was due entirely to a reduction in $^{14}CO_2$ production. Again, this suggests that the principal limiting step in glucose utilization is at the level of pyruvate oxidation.

Glucose oxidation

Direct measurements of glucose oxidation in the intact heart have been carried out by measuring $^{14}CO_2$ production from ^{14}C-glucose [24, 38] and more recently by ^{13}C-NMR spectroscopy [39]. Chen *et al.* [24] examined glucose oxidation in myocytes isolated from control, 48 hour and 4 week streptozotocin-induced diabetic rats using [U-^{14}C]glucose. As might be expected based on the earlier observations described above, they observed a marked decrease in oxidation in both diabetic groups. In the 48 hour diabetic group glucose oxidation was approximately 50-55% of control either with glucose alone (5mM) or in the presence of palmitic acid (0.4mM). With substrate concentrations that more closely mimic the *in vivo* diabetic state (i.e., elevated glucose (25mM) and palmitate (1mM)), there was a slight elevation in glucose oxidation to 65% of control values. After 4-weeks of diabetes glucose oxidation rates had decreased further to 20-25% of control values. They also examined the effect of acute insulin administration either directly to the myocytes or *in vivo* 4 hours before the experiments. In the acute diabetic group addition of insulin to the myocytes resulted in a modest but significant increase in oxidation rate and acute *in vivo* insulin administration resulted in normalization of glucose oxidation. Interestingly, in the 4-week diabetic group neither *in vitro* nor *in vivo* administration of insulin affected glucose oxidation rates. Based on these data they suggested that the metabolic alterations in the myocardium of acutely and chronically diabetic animals may represent two different diabetic states. While this may be true, it is important to note that during the first 24 hours following streptozotocin (or alloxan) treatment, there are large changes in the metabolic state of the animal [40] and it is only 24-48 hours following treatment that a new stable hyperglycemic state is reached. Thus the differences between the 48 hour and 4-week groups may simply reflect long term adaptation to the diabetic condition rather than different diabetic states.

Lopaschuk and co-workers have carried out extensive studies on the effect of diabetes on myocardial glucose oxidation [36-38]; they have principally focused on the interaction between fatty acid and glucose oxidation. In six week diabetic animals they found that glucose oxidation rates, based on $^{14}CO_2$ production from [U-^{14}C]glucose, were 8% of non-diabetic controls. As observed by Chen *et al.* [24] the addition of fatty acids decreased glucose oxidation to a similar degree in both control and diabetic groups. In 11 week diabetic animals perfused with 11 mM [U-^{14}C]glucose and 1.2mM palmitate, glucose oxidation rates normalized for differences in cardiac work were less than 5% of controls [36].

Islet cell transplantation, 3 weeks after the onset of diabetes, resulted in restoration of serum glucose to control levels. This treatment also lowered serum triglycerides, cholesterol and glycosylated hemoglobin. Glucose oxidation in the islet transplanted group was significantly improved (more that 8 fold) compared to the untreated diabetic group but was still significantly depressed compared to controls.

We have recently used ^{13}C-NMR spectroscopy to study intermediary metabolism in normal and diabetic hearts [39]. Using ^{13}C-labeled substrates intermediary metabolism can be investigated by following the incorporation of the label into different intermediates. For example, as [1-^{13}C]glucose is metabolized, the label is incorporated into the 3-carbon position in the trioses and then from the C_3-pyruvate to C_2-acetyl-CoA and subsequently into the TCA cycle intermediates. Due to the lack of sensitivity of the technique it is only possible to detect intermediates in the millimolar range; therefore as an indication of flux through glycolysis we are usually only able to detect incorporation in lactate and alanine. TCA cycle intermediates are usually below the level of detection; however, glutamate which is in rapid exchange with the TCA cycle is in the appropriate concentration range and thus we are able to follow glucose oxidation by incorporation of ^{13}C-label into glutamate. (More detail on the use of ^{13}C-NMR spectroscopy in the study of cardiac metabolism can be found in recent reviews by Malloy and co-workers [41,42])

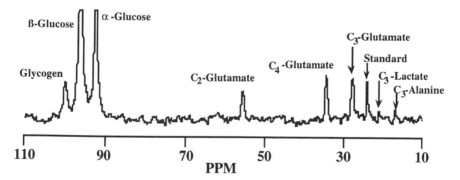

Figure 9.1 A typical ^{13}C-NMR spectrum of an isolated heart perfused for 50 minutes with [1-^{13}C]glucose as substrate.

197

A typical ^{13}C-NMR spectrum of an isolated perfused heart can been seen in Figure 9.1. Peaks from glucose, glycogen, glutamate, lactate and alanine are all visible, indicating metabolism of glucose via glycogen synthesis, glycolysis and the TCA cycle.

In a preliminary series of experiments following 1 week of streptozotocin-induced diabetes, we were unable to detect the incorporation of ^{13}C-label from [1-^{13}C]glucose (11mM) into glycogen, lactate or glutamate, consistent with a marked decrease in glucose utilization [39]. Following the addition of supra-physiological levels of insulin (0.05 units/ml) to maximally stimulate glucose transport, we observed some incorporation of label into lactate, but there was still no labeling of glutamate, indicating no oxidation of glucose. It was only following the addition of dichloroacetate (2mM), to stimulate pyruvate dehydrogenase, that label was incorporated into glutamate consistent with glucose oxidation.

High resolution ^{13}C-NMR spectroscopy of heart extracts following perfusion with ^{13}C-labeled substrates can provide detailed information regarding the relative contribution of different substrates to the TCA cycle [41]. We examined the contribution of glucose to the TCA cycle in control and 1-week diabetic animals with glucose alone, plus insulin, and with insulin plus dichloroacetate. We found that cardiac function was depressed by about 25% in the diabetic group regardless of the perfusion conditions, and there was a small but significant decrease in coronary flow. From analysis of the high resolution ^{13}C-NMR spectra we were able to determine that in the control group exogenous [1-^{13}C]glucose contributed 87±6% of the substrate entering the TCA cycle with glucose alone, 92±3% with insulin and 99±2% with glucose, insulin and dichloroacetate. In the diabetic group, glucose contributed 64±8%, 45±24% and 88±3% with glucose only, glucose plus insulin and glucose, insulin and dichloroacetate respectively. Analysis of variance confirmed that glucose oxidation was significantly depressed in the diabetic group and that dichloroacetate significantly increased the contribution of glucose to the TCA cycle. Insulin alone had no effect on glucose oxidation. Since dichloroacetate rather than insulin stimulated glucose oxidation in the diabetic heart, this provides further evidence that the principal limiting step in myocardial glucose

198

oxidation following diabetes is at the level of pyruvate dehydrogenase.

It is interesting to note that in our initial studies on the intact heart, we were unable to see any evidence of glucose oxidation in the absence of DCA, whereas in our more recent studies we were able to detect significant labeling of the glutamate pool under these conditions. This could be due in part to a 50% decrease in glutamate concentration which would significantly decrease the signal-to-noise in the spectra of the intact heart. However, in our initial experiments the hearts were allowed to beat spontaneously, whereas is the second series of experiments, hearts were paced. It has been shown that electrical stimulation results in an increase in PDH activity [43]. It is possible, therefore, that pacing itself may lead to an increase in glucose oxidation in the diabetic group.

Chen *et al.* [24] showed there was a significant decrease in glucose oxidation in isolated myocytes between 48 hours and 4 weeks of diabetes. We have also found that as the duration of diabetes increases there is a progressive decline in glucose oxidation. In hearts from six-week diabetic animals, perfused with glucose plus insulin we found that glucose contributed approximately 30-40% of the total TCA cycle flux; unlike the one-week group, the addition of dichloroacetate had no significant effect on glucose oxidation. Therefore, while in the one-week diabetic group, glucose oxidation in the presence of insulin and DCA was similar controls (88±3% of total TCA cycle flux), in the six week diabetic group, glucose contributed only 42±2% of the substrates entering the TCA cycle under the same conditions. Cardiac function was also markedly depressed in the six-week group compared to the one-week group. These results indicate that as the duration of uncontrolled diabetes increases both the functional and metabolic abnormalities become progressively worse. Furthermore, while the metabolic abnormalities are at least partially reversible after one week of diabetes, they appear to be irreversible after 6 weeks of diabetes.

The observation that the effect of diabetes on metabolism increases as the duration of diabetes increases is consistent with other studies. Data from several studies have been combined and summarized (Figure 9.2) to examine the effect of the duration of diabetes on glucose oxidation. Despite the variety of experimental models, the data is remarkably consistent and indicates that as the duration of diabetes increases, glucose oxidation rates decrease, such that after 2-3 months glucose oxidation is less than 10% of control.

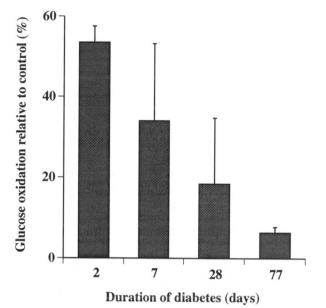

Figure 9.2: The effect of the duration of diabetes on cardiac glucose oxidation. Data summarized from several studies [24,36-38,44] including studies where glucose was the sole substrate and where palmitate was also present. It should be noted that while palmitate significantly decreased the absolute values of glucose oxidation, the effect was similar in both the control and diabetic groups and thus did not affect glucose oxidation in the diabetic groups relative to controls. Error bars represent the standard deviation of the means of the different experiments.

It is clear there is a decrease in myocardial glucose metabolism following diabetes. While some of this may be accounted for by decreased transport and phosphorylation, there is a significant decrease in glucose oxidation. It is unclear whether the alterations in transport and phosphorylation are be a consequence of the decreased rates of oxidation. There is some data to indicate that while stimulation of PDH with DCA significantly increases glucose oxidation, addition of insulin does not, which suggests that even though glucose transport and phosphorylation may be reduced following diabetes the principal limiting step in glucose utilization is at the level of glucose entry into the TCA cycle.

The effect of diabetes on pyruvate dehydrogenase

The reaction between pyruvate, CoA and NAD to form acetyl-CoA and NADH is catalyzed by a multienzyme complex located in the mitochondria -- namely the pyruvate dehydrogenase complex (PDHc). PDHc represents the principal entry point of the products of glycolysis into the TCA cycle. This complex contains three component enzymes: E_1 which catalyzes the removal of CO_2 from pyruvate and is irreversible; E_2 which forms acetyl-CoA and E_3 which reduces NAD^+ to $NADH_2$. An additional component of PDHc is a binding protein, protein X, which binds E_3 to the complex.

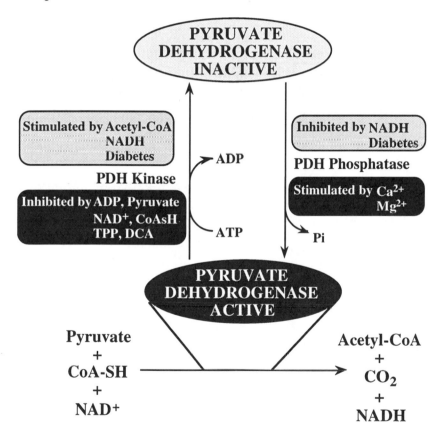

Figure 9.3: Mechanisms of regulation of PDHc activity and the effect of diabetes. TPP = thiamin pyrophosphate, coenzyme for PDHa; DCA = Dichloroacetate.

PDHc is regulated by reversible phosphorylation by two enzymes -- PDH kinase catalyzes phosphorylation of the enzyme leading to inactivation and PDH phosphatase which catalyzes dephosphorylation and reactivation. The regulation of PDH and a summary of the effects of diabetes on PDHc activity is summarized in Figure 9.3. (See [45-48] for more detail on the control and regulation of PDHc).

In the studies by Garland and colleagues [9] they observed that oxidation, of pyruvate was significantly reduced in acute uncontrolled diabetes. They also noted that fatty acids and ketone bodies had similar effects to diabetes on pyruvate oxidation. Based on these studies they concluded that diabetes resulted in the inhibition of PDHc due to an elevation in the acetyl-CoA/CoA ratio resulting from increased fatty acid and ketone body availability in the perfused heart. Subsequently it was shown that following 2 days of insulin withdrawal the active form of PDHc (PDHa) in hearts from alloxan-diabetic rats was only 10% of the total compared with 70% in non-diabetic fed rats [49]. There was also a 30% decrease in total PDHc activity in the diabetic group. These results were very similar to the effects of 24 hour starvation. The effects of diabetes were almost completely reversed by insulin treatment. By pooling data from a variety of experimental groups (i.e., treated and untreated diabetic; 24 and 48 hour starved; fasted and refed), Wieland et al. [49] showed that there was a relationship between the fraction of PDH in the active form and serum free fatty acid concentration -- above 0.5mM fatty acid, PDHa was 20% or less of the total whereas below 0.5mM, PDHa ranged from 20-80% of the total. These data suggested that serum free fatty acid levels may play a role in at least the short term regulation of PDHc activity in the heart. This is an important observation since hyper-lipidemia is usually present in diabetes.

In series of studies Kerbey and co-workers investigated the effect of diabetes on the regulation of PDH in the rat heart [50-53]. Under normal conditions with glucose and insulin as substrates, the fraction of PDHc in the active form ranged from 29% (in the absence of pyruvate) to 78% (with 25mM pyruvate). In hearts perfused with 1mM dichloroacetate, PDHa reached 95% of the total activity [50]. In contrast, following acute diabetes (40-48hrs after 60mg/kg of alloxan), PDHa was 1.5% of total activity with glucose and insulin alone, and 35.4% with the addition of DCA. In mitochondria isolated from rat hearts the total activity of PDHc was not different between diabetic and non-diabetic animals; however, the fraction in the active form and the response to pyruvate and dichloroacetate was similar to that seen in the whole heart [50]. Subsequently they showed that in mitochondria from normal hearts the fraction of PDHc in the active form was related to the ratios of ATP/ADP, NADH/NAD and acetyl-CoA/CoA. In mitochondria from diabetic hearts which had significantly reduced PDHa, they found that ATP/ADP and NADH/NAD ratios were lower compared to controls, which would tend to increase the formation of PDHa; whereas the acetyl-CoA/CoA ratio was higher than controls and would favor a decrease in PDHa. Furthermore, while pyruvate significantly increased PDHa in the diabetic group it did not alter the metabolite ratios [51]. They concluded therefore that the regulation of PDH kinase was altered in response to diabetes.

Acute alloxan diabetes as well as starvation leads to an increase in the activity of PDH kinase, resulting in the increased formation of the PDH phosphate -- the inactive form of PDHc. Hutson and Randle reported that following diabetes there was an increased rate of incorporation of ^{32}P into PDH [52] in both the presence and absence of pyruvate. This increased rate of phosphorylation corresponded to a decrease in the active form of PDHc. They also showed that in addition to an increase in the rate of phosphorylation, diabetes also resulted in a decrease in the rate of dephosphorylation and therefore reactivation [53]. These results suggest that the decreased activity of the PDHc in the heart following diabetes, is due to both an increased rate of deactivation as well as a decreased rate of reactivation. In contrast to the deactivation step, which was shown to be due to an increase in enzyme activity, the decreased rate of reactivation was not a result of a change in the phosphatase; rather it was due to a change in the PDHc phosphate. It had been previously shown that inactivation of PDHc was achieved largely (i.e., > 95%) by incorporation of only one phosphate group; an additional two phosphate groups may be incorporated. However, the fully phosphorylated complex is reactivated at approximately a third of the rate of reactivation of the partially phosphorylated complex [54-56]. It was proposed therefore that the slower reactivation of PDHc following diabetes was due to the formation of fully phosphorylated PDHc [53].

Unlike the case with hexokinase or glucose transport, diabetes does not appear to affect the total activity of PDH in the heart. Repeated studies have indicated that it is the fraction of PDH in the active form that is altered by diabetes, and it seems that this is regulated by a change in PDH kinase activity. (It should be noted that most of the studies of PDH activity following diabetes, have focused on acute diabetes (i.e., approx. 48 hours), the effects of long term diabetes on PDHc is unclear.) Starvation appears to have similar effects on PDHa and PDH kinase activity; however, the mechanism of the upregulation of PDH kinase, by starvation or diabetes is unclear. Long term regulation of enzyme activity, usually involves a change in enzyme concentration, however, this does not appear to be the case with PDH kinase. An additional protein, PDH kinase activator protein (KAP), has been isolated from the PDHc which significantly enhances PDH kinase activity. Data now suggest that KAP is the free a-subunit of PDH kinase [47,48]. Starvation leads to a greater than 2 fold increase in the V_{max} of PDH kinase in the presence of saturating KAP. Indeed the specific activity of KAP was increased 4.5 fold by starvation, yet the concentration of this protein was not significantly different following starvation. Currently there are two possible hypotheses that are consistent with the studies of starvation on the regulation of PDH kinase activity: 1) the specific activity of KAP is increased by covalent modification and 2) there are two isozymes of PDH kinase which differ in their specific activity, with starvation increasing the concentration of the more active form [47,48]. Much of the recent work on the regulation of PDH kinase activity has focused on the effects of starvation on PDH kinase in the liver. It remains to be determined whether similar changes occur in the heart during diabetes.

Diabetes and cardiac metabolism in humans

While there have been extensive investigations into cardiac metabolism in experimental models of diabetes, there is limited information on cardiac metabolism in diabetic patients. In one of the earlier studies of human myocardial metabolism, Ungar *et al.*

[57] reported that myocardial glucose extraction was depressed in diabetic patients. This observation was consistent with the study by Goodale et al. [58], who showed that glucose extraction was negligible in fasting, mildly diabetic subjects (0-6%) whereas in normal subjects it ranged from 13-31%, despite a more than 2 fold higher level of serum glucose in the diabetic group. They also reported that the percent extraction of both lactate and pyruvate were also depressed in the diabetic group. Administration of insulin normalized the extraction of glucose, lactate and pyruvate in a diabetic patient.

More recently, Avogaro et al. [59] examined arteriovenous differences of glucose, lactate, pyruvate, ketone bodies and fatty acids in 12 normal and 11 insulin dependent diabetic patients. Care was taken to ensure that the diabetics were free from coronary artery disease and had normal cardiac function both at rest and following both treadmill exercise and dipyridamole. Despite hyperglycemia, there was decreased glucose uptake in the diabetic group. Interestingly, while there was net uptake of pyruvate and lactate in controls, there was net release of these substrates in the diabetic group. Concomitant with the decrease in glucose uptake in the diabetics, there was an increase in extraction of both ketone bodies and free fatty acids. Atrial pacing stimulated glucose, lactate and pyruvate uptake in the diabetic patients such that the calculated flux rates of pyruvate into lactate and lactate into pyruvate were similar to controls. They also examined arterio-venous differences in patients during insulin withdrawal (i.e., hyperglycemia) and following insulin infusion (i.e., euglycemia) and found that under euglycemic conditions the patterns of substrate uptake and release were similar to non-diabetic controls. They concluded that the metabolic alterations observed in the diabetic group were not due to alterations in myocardial perfusion or a result of coronary artery disease. They also suggested that in their study group the presence of coronary microangiopathy was unlikely and could not account for the observed results. They concluded that the alteration in cardiac metabolism in the diabetic patients were a consequence of hypoinsulinemia and hyper-glycemia.

Positron emission tomography (PET) has recently been used to investigate myocardial glucose uptake in non-insulin dependent diabetics (NIDDM) [60] and in insulin-dependent diabetes (IDDM) [61]. Both studies emphasized the use of the insulin clamp technique to minimize differences in the metabolic state between the control and patient groups. In the NIDDM study, while whole body and skeletal muscle glucose disposal rates were similar between diabetics and nondiabetics, myocardial glucose disposal rates in diabetic patients were 39% lower than the nondiabetic group [60]. It should be noted that in all subjects had evidence of coronary artery disease although left ventricular function was normal. There was no data presented regarding the severity of the coronary artery disease; thus it cannot be ruled out that the differences in glucose uptake between the two patient groups could be due to differences in coronary artery disease.

Vom Dahl *et al.* [61], examined 9 normal and 7 insulin dependent young males. Care was taken to exclude any subjects with evidence of heart disease or hypertension. In the diabetic group all subjects had a history of diabetes for less than five years and patients with known microangiopathy were excluded. There were no baseline differences between the two groups in either hemodynamics or plasma substrate levels. In contrast to the study on NIDDM [60], vom Dahl and co-workers found no differences in glucose uptake in the diabetic subjects. It is worth emphasizing that in this study vom Dahl focused on a tightly controlled and carefully selected population of young patients that had been diabetic for only a short period of time (i.e., <5years) and as the authors noted, this group did not represent the "typical" diabetic patient.

Conclusion

Diabetes has profound effects on myocardial glucose metabolism, characterized by decreased glucose uptake; this is the case across a wide range of models of diabetes as well as in diabetic patients. This decrease in glucose uptake can be accounted for by a decrease in glucose transport, glucose phosphorylation, glucose oxidation and glycogen synthesis. These changes appear to become progressively worse as the duration of diabetes progresses, this is particularly evident in the case of glucose oxidation. The effects of diabetes on glycolysis (i.e., glucose metabolism from glucose 6-

phosphate to pyruvate and lactate) are less clear, although data suggests that it is less affected than glucose oxidation. The regulation of PDHc, which controls the entry of glucose into the TCA cycle, is significantly altered by diabetes, with an increase in PDH kinase activity leading to a decrease of PDH in the active form. Stimulation of PDHc activity with dichloroacetate significantly increases glucose oxidation in diabetic hearts. In contrast, insulin stimulates glucose transport and phosphorylation, but does not appear to increase glucose oxidation. These combined data suggests that the principal rate limiting step in glucose oxidation is at the level of PDHc rather than glucose transport or phosphorylation. This also raises the interesting question as to whether the decreases in glucose transport and phosphorylation could be secondary to the decreased flux through PDHc?

Acknowledgments

This work was supported in part by a Grant-in-Aid from the American Heart Association with funds contributed in part by the AHA, Maryland Affiliate and Grant HL 48789 from the National Institutes of Health

References

1. Leyden E. Asthma und diabetes mellitus. *Zeitschr. Kiln. Med.* **3**: 358-364, 1881.

2. Mayer J. Ueber den zusammenhang des diabetes mellitus mit erkrankungen des herzens. *Zeitschr. Klin. Med.* **14**: 209-254, 1888.

3. Knowlton FP and Starling EH. *J. Physiol. (Lond.)* **45**: 1912.

4. Cruickshank EWH. Cardiac Metabolism. *Physiol. Rev.* **16**: 597, 1936.

5. Morgan HE, Henderson MJ, Regen DM and Park CR. Regulation of glucose uptake in muscle I. The effects of insulin and anoxia on glucose transport and phosphorylation in the

isolated perfused heart of normal rats. *J. Biol. Chem.* **236**: 253-261, 1961.

6. Morgan HE, Cadenas E, Regen DM and Park CR. Regulation of glucose uptake in muscle II. Rate limiting steps and effects of insulin and anoxia in heart muscle from diabetic rats. *J. Biol. Chem.* **236**: 262-268, 1961.

7. Morgan HE, Regen DM, Henderson MJ, Sawyer TK and Park CR. Regulation of glucose uptake in muscle VI. Effects of hypophysectomy, adrenalectomy, growth hormone, hydrocortisone and insulin on glucose transport and phosphorylation in the perfused rat heart. *J. Biol. Chem.* **236**: 2162-2168, 1961.

8. Newsholme EA and Randle PJ. Regulation of glucose uptake by muscle. 7: Effects of fatty acids, ketone bodies and pyruvate, and of alloxan-diabetes, starvation, hypophysectomy and adrenalectomy, on the concentrations of hexose phosphates, nucleotides and inorganic phosphate in perfused rat heart. *Biochem. J.* **93**: 641-651, 1964.

9. Garland PB, Newsholme EA and Randle PJ. Regulation of glucose uptake by muscle. 9: Effects of fatty acids, ketone bodies and of alloxan-diabetes and starvation, on pyruvate metabolism and on lactate/pyruvate and l-glycerol 3-phosphate/dihydroxyacetone phosphate concentration ratios in rat heart and rat diaphragm muscles. *Biochem. J.* **93**: 664-678, 1964.

10. Randle PJ, Garland PB, Hales CN and Newsholme EA. The glucose fatty-acid cycle: Its role in insulin sensitivity and metabolic disturbances of diabetes mellitus. *The Lancet* **1**: 785-789, 1963.

11. Garland PB and Randle PJ. Regulation of glucose uptake by muscle. 10: Effects of alloxan-diabetes, starvation, hypophysectomy and adrenalectomy and of fatty acids, ketone bodies and pyruvate, on the glycerol output and concentrations of free fatty acids, long chain fatty acyl-coenzyme A, glycerol phosphate and citrate-cycle intermediates in rat heart and diaphragm muscles. *Biochem. J.* **93**: 678-687, 1964.

12. Randle PJ, Newsholme EA and Garland PB. Regulation of glucose uptake by muscle. 8: Effects of fatty acids, ketone bodies and pyruvate, and of alloxan-diabetes and starvation, on the uptake and metabolic fate of glucose in rat heart and diaphtagm muscles. *Biochem. J.* **93**: 652-665, 1964.

13. Post RL, Morgan HE and Park CR. Regulation of glucose uptake in muscle III. The interaction of membrane transport and phosphorylation in the control of glucose uptake. *J. Biol. Chem.* **236**: 269-272, 1961.

14. Slieker L, Sundell KL, Heath WF, Osborne E, Bue J, Manetta J and Sportsman JR. Glucose transporter levels in tissues of spontaneously diabetic zucker *fa/fa* rat (ZDF/drt) and viable yellow mouse (Avy/a). *Diabetes* **41**: 187-193, 1992.

15. Stanley WC, Hall JL, Smith KR, Cartee GD, Hacker TA and Wisneski JA. Myocardial glucose transporters and glycolytic metabolism during ischemia in hyperglycemic diabetic swine. *Metabolism* **43**: 61-69, 1994.

16. Kainulainen H, Breiner M, Schurmann A, Marttinen A, Virjo A and Joost HG. In vivo glucose uptake and glucose transporter proteins glut1 and glut4 in heart and various types of skeletal muscle from Streptozotocin-Diabetic rats. *Biochim. Biophys. Acta* **1225**: 275-282, 1994.

17. Eckel J and Reinauer H. Insulin action on glucose transport in isolated cardiac myocytes: signalling pathways and diabetes-induced alterations. *Biochem. Soc. Trans.* **18**: 1125-1127, 1990.

18. Burcelin R, Printz RL, Kande J, Assan R, Granner DK and Girard J. Regulation of glucose transporter and hexokinase II expression in tissues of diabetic rats. *Am. J. Physiol.* **265**: E392-E401, 1993.

19. Camps M, Castello A, Munoz P, Monfar M, Testar X, Palacin M and Zorzano A. Effect of diabetes and fasting on GLUT-4 (muscle/fat) glucose-transporter expression in insulin-sensitive tissues. *Biochem. J.* **282**: 765-772, 1992.

20. Garvey WT, Hardin D, Juhasova M and Dominguez JH. Effects of diabetes on myocardial glucose transport system in

rats: implications for diabetic cardiomyopathy. *Am. J. Physiol.* **264**: H837-H844, 1993.

21. Kahn BB, Rossetti L, Lodish HF and Charron MJ. Decreased in vivo glucose uptake but normal expression of GLUT1 and GLUT4 in skeletal muscle in diabetic rats. *J. Clin. Invest.* **87**: 2197-2206, 1991.

22. Klip A, Marette A, Dimitrankoudis D, Ramlal T, Giacca A, Shi ZQ, and Vranic M. Effect of diabetes on glucoregulation. From glucose transporters to glucose metabolism in vivo. *Diabetes Care* **15**: 1747-1766, 1992.

23. England PJ and Randle PJ. Effectors of rat-heart hexokinase and the control of glucose phosphorylation in the perfused rat heart. *Biochem. J.* **105**: 907-920, 1967.

24. Chen V, Ianuzzo CD, Fong BC and Spitzer JJ. The effects of acute and chronic diabetes on myocardial metabolism in rats. *Diabetes* **33**: 1078-1084, 1984.

25. Sochor M, Kunjara S, Ali M and McLean P. Vanadate treatment increases the activity of glycolytic enzymes and raises fructose 2,6-bisphosphate concentration in hearts from diabetic rats. *Biochem. Int.* **28**: 525-531, 1992.

26. Katzen HM. The multiple forms of mammalian hexokinase and their significance to the action of insulin. *Advan. Enzyme Regul.* **5**: 335-356, 1967.

27. Sochor M, Baquer NZ, Hothersall JS and McLean P. Effect of experimental diabetes on the activity of hexokinase isoenzymes in tissues of the rat. *Biochem. Int.* **22**: 467-474, 1990.

28. Katzen HM, Soderman DD and Wiley CE. Multiple forms of hexokinase. Activities associated with subcellular particulate and soluble fractions of normal and streptozotocin diabetic rat tissues. *J. Biol. Chem.* **245**: 4081-4096, 1970.

29. Anderson JW and Stowring L. Glycolytic and gluconeogenic enzyme activities in renal cortex of diabetic rats. *Am. J. Physiol.* **224**: 930-936, 1973.

30. Regen DM, Davies WW and Morgan HE. *Fed. Proc.* **20**: 83, 1961.

31. Newshome EA and Randle PJ. Regulation of glucose uptake by muscle. 5. Effects of anoxia, insulin, adrenalin and prolonged starving on concentrations of hexose phosphates in isolated rat diaphragam and perfused isolated rat heart. *Biochem J.* **80**: 655-662, 1961.

32. Newshome EA and Randle PJ. Regulation of glucose uptake by muscle. 6. Fructose 1,6-diphosphate activity of rat heart and rat diaphragm. *Biochem. J.* **83**: 387-392, 1962.

33. Newsholme EA, Randle PJ and Manchester KL. Inhibition of the phosphofructokinase reaction in perfused rat heart by respiration of ketone bodies,fatty acids and pyruvate. *Nature* **193**: 270, 1962.

34. Chen V and Ianuzzo CD. Dosage effect of streptozotocin on rat tissue enzyme activities and glycogen content. *Can. J. Physiol. Pharmacol.* **60**: 1251-1256, 1982.

35. Opie LH, Mansford KRL and Owen P. Effects of increased heart work on glycolysis and adenine nucleotides in the perfused heart of normal and diabetic rats. *Biochem. J.* **124**: 475-490, 1971.

36. Lopaschuk GD, Lakey JRT, Barr R, Wambolt R, Thomson ABR, Clandinin MT and Rajotte RV. Islet transplantation improves glucose oxidation and mechanical function in diabetic rat hearts. *Can J Physiol Pharmacol* **71**: 896-903, 1993.

37. Gamble J and Lopaschuk GD. Glycolysis and glucose oxidation during reperfusion of ischemic hearts from diabetic rats. *Biochim. Biophys. Acta* **1225**: 191-199, 1994.

38. Wall SR and Lopaschuk GD. Glucose oxidation rates in fatty acid-perfused isolated working hearts from diabetic rats. *Biochim. Biophys. Acta* **1006**: 97-103, 1989.

39. Chatham JC and Forder JR. A ^{13}C-NMR study of glucose oxidation in the intact functioning rat heart following diabetes-induced cardiomyopathy. *J. Mol. Cell. Cardiol.* **25**: 1203-1213, 1993.

40. Pierce GN, Beamish RE and Dhalla NS. *Heart Dysfunction in Diabetes*. Boca Raton, FL.: CRC Press, 1988.

41. Malloy CR, Sherry AD and Jeffrey FMH. Analysis of tricarboxylic acid cycle of the heart using ^{13}C isotope isomers. *Am. J. Physiol.* **259**: H987-H995, 1990.

42. Sherry AD and Malloy CR. Cardiac metabolism. In RJ Gillies (Eds.), *"NMR in Physiology and Biomedicine"* (pp. 439-449). 525 B Street, Suite 1900, San Diego, CA 92101-4495: Academic Press Inc, 1994.

43. Hansford RG, Hogue B, Prokopczuk A, Wasilewska E and Lewartowski B. Activation of pyruvate dehydrogenase by electrical stimulation, and low Na^+ perfusion of guinea-pig heart. *Biochim. Biophys. Acta* **1018**: 282-286, 1990.

44. Rosen P, Windeck P, Zimmer H-G, Frenzel H, Burrig KF and Reinauer H. Myocardial performance and metabolism in non-ketotic, diabetic rat hearts: myocardial function and metabolism in vivo and in the isolated perfused heart under the influence of insulin and octanoate. *Bas. Res. Cardiol.* **81**: 620-635, 1986.

45. Reed LJ. Regulation of mammalian pyruvate dehydrogenase complex by a phosphorylation -dephosphorylation cycle. *Curr. Top. Cell. Regul.* **18**: 95-106, 1981.

46. Randle PJ. Fuel selection in animals. Nineteenth Ciba Medal Lecture. *Biohcem. Soc. Trans.* **14**: 799-806, 1986.

47. Randle PJ, Priestman DA, Mistry S and Halsall A. Mechanisms modifying glucose oxidation in diabetes mellitus. *Diabetologia* **37**: S155-S161, 1994.

48. Randle PJ, Priestman DA, Mistry SC and Halsall A. Glucose fatty acid interactions and the regulation of glucose disposal. *J Cell Biochem* **55**: 1-11, 1994.

49. Wieland O, Siess E, Schulze-Wethmar FH, van Funcke HG and Winton B. Active and inactive forms of pyruvate dehydrogenase in rat heart and kidney: effect of diabetes, fasting and refeeding on pyruvate dehydrogenase interconversion. *Arch. Biochem. Biophys.* **143**: 593-601, 1971.

50. Kerbey AL, Randle PJ, Cooper RH, Whitehouse S, PAsk HT and Denton RM. Mechanism of regulation of proportions of deposphorylated and phosphorylated enzyme by oxidation of

fatty acids and ketone bodies and of effects of diabetes: role of coenzyme A, acetyl-coA and reduced and oxidized nicotinamide-adenine dinucleotide. *Biochem. J.* **154**: 327-348, 1976.

51. Kerbey AL, Radcliff PM and Randle PJ. Diabetes and the control of pyruvate dehydrogenase in rat heart mitochondria by concentration ratios of adenosine triphosphate/adenosine diphosphate, of reduced/oxidized nicotinamide-adenine di-nucleotide and of acetyl-coenzyme A/coenzyme A. *Biochem. J.* **64**: 509-519, 1977.

52. Hutson NJ and Randle PJ. Enhanced activity of pyruvate dehydrogenase kinase in rat heart mitochondria in alloxan-diabetes or starvation. *FEBS Lett.* **92**: 73-76, 1978.

53. Hutson NJ, Kerbey AL, Randle PJ and Sugden PH. Conversion of inactive (phosphorylated) pyruvate dehydrogenase complex into active complex by the phosphate reaction in heart mitochondria is inhibited by alloxan-diabetes or starvation. *Biochem. J.* **173**: 669-680, 1978.

54. Sugden PH, Hutson NJ, Kerbey AL and Randle PJ. Phosphorylation of additional sites on pyruvate dehydrogenase inhibits its reactivation by pyruvate dehydrogenase phosphate phosphatase. *Biochem. J.* **168,** 1979.

55. Sugden PH and Randle PJ. Regulation of pig heart pyruvate dehydrogenase by phosphorylation studies on the subunit and phosphorylation stoicheiometries. *Biochem. J.* **173**: 659-668, 1978.

56. Davis PF, Pettit FH and Reed LJ. Peptides derived from pyruvate dehydrogenase as substrates for pyruvate dehydrogenase kinase and phosphatase. *Biochem. Biophys. Res. Commun.* **75**: 541-549, 1977.

57. Ungar I, Gilbert M, Siegal A, Blair JM and Bing RJ. Studies on myocardial metabolism. *Am. J. Med.* **18**: 385-396, 1955.

58. Goodale WT, Olson RE and Hackel DB. The effects of fasting and diabetes mellitus on myocardial metabolism in man. *Am. J. Med.* **27**: 212-220, 1959.

59. Avogaro A, Nosadini R, Doria A, Fioretto P, Velussi M, Vigorito C, Sacca L, Toffolo G, C. C, Trevisan R, Duner E, Razzolini R, Rengo F and Crepaldi G. Myocardial metabolism in insulin-deficient diabetic humans without coronary artery disease. *Am. J. Physiol.* **258**: E606-E618, 1990.

60. Voipio-Pulkki L-M, Nuutila P, Knuutti MJ, Ruotsalainen U, Haaparanta M, Teras M, Wegelius U and Koivisto VA. Heart and skeletal muscle disposal in type 2 diabetic patients as determined by positron emission tomography. *J. Nucl. Med.* **34**: 2064-2076, 1993.

61. vom Dahl J, Herman WH, Hicks RJ, Ortiz-Alonso FJ, Lee KS, Allman KC, Wolfe ER, Kalff V and Schwaiger M. Myocardial glucose uptake in patients with insulin-dependent diabetes mellitus assessed quatitatively by dynamic positron emission tomography. *Circulation* **88**: 395-404, 1993.

CHAPTER 10

Fatty Acid Metabolism in the Heart Following Diabetes

Gary D. Lopaschuk

Introduction

Under normal physiological conditions the heart uses a combination of carbohydrates and fatty acids as a fuel source, with fatty acid oxidation typically providing 60 to 70% of the heart's energy needs [1-5]. In uncontrolled diabetes, carbohydrate use decreases and fatty acid oxidation can provide from 90 to 100 % of the heart's ATP requirements [3,6-9]. While decreased glucose uptake due to insulin deficiency can partly explain the decrease in glucose metabolism, classic studies from Sir Philip Randle's laboratory have demonstrated that fatty acids are primarily responsible for the decrease in glycolysis and glucose oxidation in the diabetic heart [6,7,10-13]. Plasma free fatty acid levels are elevated in patients with either non-insulin dependent or insulin-dependent diabetes [15], and are thought to play a major role in the development of fasting hyperglycemia [14,15,16]. While high levels of fatty acids inhibits glycolysis, they also result in a marked inhibition of the pyruvate dehydrogenase complex [7,11,13,14], resulting in a marked decrease in glucose oxidation [9,17-20]. This is primarily due to activation of pyruvate dehydrogenase kinase, secondary to an increase in the intramitochondrial acetyl CoA/CoA ratio [6,7,10-13].

Although high circulating levels of fatty acids in the diabetic can decrease glucose metabolism, it is clear that other metabolic changes in the heart are also responsible for low glucose oxidation rates. For instance, the decrease in pyruvate dehydrogenase complex activity seen in diabetic rat hearts exceeds what would be expected if the inhibition occurred solely due to high levels of fatty acids [13]. This is supported by the observation that glucose oxidation rates are significantly lower in diabetic rat hearts compared to control hearts, even if hearts are perfused with similar concentrations of fatty acids [6,17,20]. As will be discussed, we believe that this is due, in part, to an alteration in the regulation of fatty acid oxidation in the diabetic heart.

In the last decade it has also become clear that alterations in fatty acid metabolism contribute to a depression in contractile function that has been well characterized in the diabetic (i.e. diabetic cardiomyopathy). Experimental studies have demonstrated that a decrease in carbohydrate metabolism and an increased reliance of the heart on fatty acids as an energy source contribute to the severity of diabetic cardiomyopathies. It has also become apparent that alterations in fatty acid metabolism alter the outcome of ischemic injury in the diabetic. The possible mechanisms responsible for this will be discussed.

Relationship between fatty acid and glucose metabolism

The heart has a tight coupling between carbohydrate and fatty acid metabolism. Glucose and lactate are the important carbohydrates utilized, while free fatty acids (predominantly oleic acid and palmitic acid) are the key lipids oxidized. Although ketone bodies and amino acids can be utilized by the heart, neither is a major substrate under normal aerobic conditions. In severe ketotic diabetes, ketones can become an important fuel of the heart, although oxidation of these short chain carbon substrates are not normally a significant source of ATP production in the heart. (See Chaper 7 for more details on ketone body metabolism in the heart.)

As mentioned, a key determinant of glucose utilization is the level of circulating fatty acids [3,5,15,21-23]. In diabetics, in which plasma levels of both free fatty acids and triacylglycerol-rich lipoproteins increase, fatty acid inhibition of both glycolysis and

Table 10.1: Comparison of cardiac fatty acid and glucose oxidation rates in various animals models of diabetes

Animal Model	Fatty Acid Oxidation	Glucose Oxidation	Reference
Streptozotocin Diabetic Rats			
-uncontrolled	normal	decreased	9,17, 28,29
-islet transplanted	normal	normal	30,31
Spontaneously Diabetic BB Rats			
-controlled	normal	normal	32,33
-uncontrolled	increased	decreased	
Insulin-resistant JCR/LA rat			
-high insulin	normal	normal	34,35
-low insulin	unknown	unknown	

In all of the studies listed above, comparison between diabetic and control hearts were performed under similar perfusion conditions (i.e., identical levels of fatty acids in the perfusate). In most of the studies listed above a significant depression of heart function was observed in uncontrolled diabetic rat hearts. As a result, the amount of fatty acid oxidized per unit of work was actually accelerated in these hearts.

glucose oxidation in the heart is especially prominent. As a result, the heart can become almost entirely dependent on fatty acid oxidation to meet its energy requirements [9,24].

Early studies in humans have shown that glucose uptake is markedly decreased in diabetics [8] with an increased extraction of fatty acids [25]. In experimental animal studies the uptake [25,26] of free fatty acids is either normal or accelerated. In contrast, Kreisberg has demonstrated that uptake and oxidation of fatty acids originating from chylomicrons is decreased in diabetic rat hearts [27]. This same study suggested that endogenous triacylglycerol turnover was increased in the diabetic rat heart (as discussed later). Although oxidation of fatty acid originating from lipoproteins may be depressed in diabetes, it is clear the oxidation of circulating free fatty acids is not decreased. Measurement of fatty acid oxidation in hearts obtained from a number of different animals models of diabetes have shown that fatty acid oxidation is either unchanged or increased (Table 10.1). In fact, if alterations in contractile function are considered, fatty acid oxidation normalized for cardiac work can be accelerated in the diabetic rat heart.

Alterations in fatty acid oxidation

Circulating fatty acids and lipoproteins
The main source of fatty acids for the heart are free fatty acids bound to albumin, and fatty acid esters present in chylomicrons and very low density lipoproteins (VLDL). In diabetics, levels of both free fatty acids and circulating lipoproteins are elevated [14, 36]. While high circulating levels of fatty acids increases the contribution of fatty acids as a source of ATP production in the diabetic heart, the effects of elevated levels of lipoproteins on myocardial fatty acid metabolism is not clear. Earlier studies by Kreisberg showed that oxidation of chylomicron fatty acids is decreased in diabetic rat hearts [27]. This may be due to a decrease in lipoprotein lipase (LPL) activity, the enzyme responsible for the release of fatty acids from triacylglycerol contained in chylomicrons and VLDL. While earlier studies have suggested that LPL activity is increased in streptozotocin diabetic rat hearts [37,38], recent studies by Severson's laboratory have shown a diabetes-induced reduction in heart LPL activity [39-41]. Isolated perfused hearts from steptozotocin diabetic rats have a decrease in heparin-releasable LPL activity [39-41]. Decreased LPL activity may, in part, be due to an inhibitory effect of free fatty acids [40], which are elevated in the diabetic.

As a result, it appears that while metabolism of free fatty acids is high in the diabetic heart, the metabolism of fatty acids esterified to lipoproteins is decreased. However, this issue is complicated by the fact that the relative proportion of fatty acids used by the heart that are derived from either free fatty acids or fatty acids esterified in lipoprotein triacylglycerols has yet to be determined.

Transport of fatty acids into the myocytes

The transport of fatty acids across (or around) the endothelial cells, across the interstitial space, and subsequently across the sarcolemmal membrane is presently a source of debate [see ref. 42 for review]. At the level of the sarcolemmal membrane controversy also exists as to whether fatty acids are taken up by simple diffusion or a carrier mediated process (see ref. 42 for discussion of this issue). Until this issue is resolved, it is not clear whether diabetes induced changes in these transport or uptake processes contribute to the high rates of fatty acid oxidation in the diabetic heart.

Once inside the aqueous cytoplasm fatty acids bind to heart-type fatty acid binding proteins (FABPs). FABPs are a class of low molecular weight (14-15 kDa) proteins, which are highly abundant in tissues which actively metabolize fatty acids, and are capable of binding hydrophobic ligands [see ref. 42 for review]. Heart type FABP is among the most abundant of cardiac proteins, comprising about 2% of the soluble cytoplasmic proteins [43]. Compelling evidence for a role of FABPs in fatty acid metabolism comes from the high correlation between the content of FABPs in various tissues and the capacity of these tissues to oxidize palmitate under a variety of pathological or pharmacological conditions [44]. In hearts from both insulin-dependent and non-insulin-dependent diabetic rats cardiac FABP increases dramatically compared to age matched controls [45]. The increase in FABP content may either adapt to or enable a higher rate of fatty acid utilization by the diabetic heart. However, it has yet to be established whether altered FABP content is a cause or consequence of the high rates of fatty acid metabolism.

The conversion of the carboxylic head group of fatty acids to the more reactive CoA thioester (a process known as fatty acid activation), is a prerequisite for the subsequent catabolic processes. This conversion of fatty acids to their acyl-CoA esters is catalyzed by a family of acyl-CoA synthetases which differ in their chain length specificity and their subcellular location [46]. In the heart, long-chain acyl-CoA synthetase is localized to the aqueous cytoplasmic face of the mitochondrial membrane [46]. Acyl CoA then presumably binds to an acyl CoA binding protein [47]. Despite the obligatory role for the acyl CoA synthetases in the catabolic pathway of fatty acids, their regulatory influence on fatty acid metabolism has yet to be completely elucidated [48]. While recent studies have shown that acyl CoA synthetase expression can change under conditions of altered fatty acid metabolism, the effects of diabetes on acyl CoA synthetase activity and expression have not been determined.

A better understanding of acyl-CoA synthetase activity in the diabetic heart is important, since a number of previous studies have implicated accumulation of long chain acyl CoA as contributing to contractile dysfunction [see ref. 49 for review]. Long chain acyl CoA are amphiphilic compounds that have the potential to alter the activity of a number of membrane enzymes. Long chain acyl CoAs are also potent inhibitors of the mitochondrial adenine nucleotide transporter [50]. It has been suggested that accumulation of long chain acyl CoA esters in the diabetic rat heart will result in a decrease in ATP levels [51], although this has not been confirmed in other studies.

Mitochondrial uptake of fatty acids

Once activated in the aqueous cytoplasm, long-chain acyl-CoAs are transferred into the mitochondrial matrix by the concerted efforts of three carnitine-dependent enzymes. The first of these enzymes, carnitine palmitoyl transferase-1 (CPT-1), catalyzes the formation of long-chain acylcarnitine to form long-chain acyl-CoA. The topography of this enzyme has been a source of great debate, although it is now generally accepted that it is located on the inner surface of the outer mitochondrial membrane [52]. The second enzyme, carnitine:acylcarnitine translocase transports long-chain acylcarnitine across the inner mitochondrial membrane. The third enzyme, CPT-2, is associated with the inner mitochondrial membrane and catalyzes the reverse reaction ultimately regenerating long-chain acyl-CoA within the mitochondrial matrix.

Long-chain acylcarnitines formed by CPT-1 are preferentially transported into mitochondria despite the presence of much higher concentrations of extra mitochondrial free-carnitine and short-chain acylcarnitine. This is because affinity of carnitine:acylcarnitine translocase for extra mitochondrial acylcarnitine is much higher than for external carnitine and short-chain acylcarnitine [53,54]. The translocase activity is determined by free carnitine concentrations in the mitochondrial matrix [54]. The carnitine concentration in the mitochondrial matrix is also determined by the translocase, which catalyzes a slow transport of carnitine [55]. Studies indicate that liver and heart mitochondria contain sufficient translocase activity such that the translocase is not the rate-limiting step in the carnitine transport [56]. However, studies in the isolated rat heart have suggested that the translocase step limits the rate of fatty acid oxidation at high levels of ventricular pressure development [57].

CPT-1 is the key regulatory enzyme involved in the mitochondrial uptake of fatty acids. This enzyme transfers the fatty acid moiety from acyl-CoA to carnitine forming long chain acyl-carnitine, which is then transported into the mitochondria [see ref. 58 for review]. Malonyl-CoA, which is produced by acetyl-CoA carboxylase (ACC), is a potent inhibitor of CPT-1 [59,60], and acts at a site distinct from the catalytic site of CPT-1, which may be a distinct malonyl CoA binding protein [61,62] or at a site on CPT-1 itself [52,59,60,63-66]. Recent cloning of liver CPT-1 has shown that molecular weight of CPT-1 is 88 kDa [64,67]. This isoform is also present in heart, although an 82 kDa isoform of CPT-1 appears to predominate [68]. The 82 kDa CPT-1 is thought to be most sensitive to inhibition by malonyl CoA [68].

In liver the IC_{50} of CPT-1 for malonyl CoA increases dramatically in diabetes [60,63,69-72]. As a result, higher concentrations of malonyl CoA are required to inhibit fatty acid oxidation and, theoretically, malonyl CoA becomes less important as a regulator of hepatic fatty acid oxidation. In heart, CPT-1 is much more sensitive to malonyl CoA inhibition than liver, with CPT-1 having an IC_{50} for malonyl CoA in the 30-50 nM range [60,68,73]. Furthermore, in contrast to liver, the sensitivity of heart CPT-1 to malonyl CoA inhibition does not change in diabetic animals [74]. In a number of other conditions in which fatty acid oxidation widely varies we have also observed that the IC_{50} of mitochondrial CPT-1 for malonyl CoA also does not change [75,76]. Accumulating evidence suggests that actual changes in malonyl CoA levels appear to be the key factor regulating changes in fatty acid oxidation in the heart, as opposed to changes in sensitivity of CPT-1 to malonyl CoA inhibition. The key enzyme responsible for malonyl CoA production in the heart is acetyl CoA carboxylase.

Regulation of fatty acid oxidation by acetyl CoA carboxylase

Acetyl-coenzyme A carboxylase (ACC) is best known as the rate-limiting enzyme in fatty acid biosynthesis in liver and adipose tissue [77-79]. In the heart ACC is also present, despite the fact that the heart has a very low capacity for fatty acid synthesis [80-85]. Two isoforms of ACC are expressed, a 280 kDa isoform (which predominates) and a 265 kDa isoform. Studies from our laboratory [80-85] and others [86] suggest that ACC in the heart functions primarily as a regulator of fatty acid oxidation, due to inhibition of CPT 1 by malonyl-CoA. In other tissues ACC also appears to have functions other than fatty acid biosynthesis. Recent studies in pancreatic islet cells have suggested that malonyl CoA production may have an important role in glucose-stimulated insulin secretion [86-88]. Inhibition of CPT-1 by malonyl CoA is thought to increase acyl CoA levels, which trigger insulin release.

The liver 265 kDa ACC has been shown to be regulated in two different time frames, a rapid regulation (minutes) and a long term regulation (hours/days) [77,79,80,90-95]. The long term regulation of ACC involves tissue-specific use of diverse ACC gene promoters, and changes in the rate of transcription, synthesis and degradation of ACC. The rapid regulation of ACC occurs due to both covalent phosphorylation and allosteric regulation [79,80]. Although the regulation of the 265 kDa isoform has been extensively studied in the liver, little is known about regulation of the ACC in the heart, in which the 280 kDa isoform predominates. It is apparent that cytoplasmic acetyl CoA supply to ACC is one mechanism of control [82,83], although it is now becoming clear that phosphorylation control of the enzyme is also important in the regulation of heart ACC [85].

In recent experiments we have investigated diabetes induced changes in ACC expression and activity in hearts obtained from streptozotocin diabetic rats [85]. Despite the presence of severe diabetes, neither the levels of mRNA for the 280 kDa isoform of ACC or the protein expression of either the 280 kDa or 265 kDa isoform were altered. However, a significant depression of ACC activity was seen. These results suggest that the primary change in ACC activity in diabetic rat hearts occurs due to an alteration in either phosphorylation control or allosteric control, as opposed to an alteration in expression of ACC. This contrasts the liver and adipose tissue, in which we observed a dramatic decrease in ACC expression in diabetic animals.

Regulation of ACC activity

Although a number of different kinases will phosphorylate the 265 kDa isoform of ACC (ACC-265) *in vitro*, it is now apparent that cAMP-dependent protein kinase and a recently characterized 5'AMP activated protein kinase (AMPK) are the kinases important in regulating liver ACC activity [96,97]. Phosphorylation of ser-1200 of ACC-265 by cAMP-dependent protein kinase results in inactivation of the 265 kDa isoform of liver ACC, and is thought to be one of the mechanisms by which glucagon inhibits ACC [90, 92]. A recent study by Wins *et al.* [98] has shown that the 280 kDa isoform of liver ACC can also be phosphorylated by cAMP-dependent protein kinase. Whether this results in an inactivation of ACC activity has not been determined. Although cAMP-dependent protein kinase can directly phosphorylate ACC, recent studies by Hardie have suggested that cAMP-dependent protein kinase in the liver may act primarily through activation of AMPK [96, 97].

Table 10.2: Activity of 5'AMP activated protein kinase (AMPK) and acetyl CoA carboxylase in insulin resistant JCR/LA corpulent rat hearts

	AMPK Activity (pmol/min/mg)	ACC Activity (nmol/min/mg)
Lean control	272 ± 35	36.67 ± 12.34
Insulin-resistant	$499 \pm 52*$	$14.41 \pm 5.62*$

*Values are means $\pm$ S.E. of 5 hearts in each group. (AMPK, 5'AMP activated protein kinase: ACC, acetyl CoA carboxylase). AMPK and ACC were measured in heart extracts as described in references 30, 80, 82, 85. * = significantly different than lean control.*

In liver, AMPK functions to conserve energy by inhibiting anabolic processes when cellular ATP levels are depleted and AMP levels increase [96]. We have recently optimized conditions for measurement of AMPK activity in heart tissue, and found that this activity exceeds the activity observed in liver. This is supported by recent work in Witters laboratory that has shown that AMPK mRNA levels in heart exceed levels seen in liver (Gao and Witters, personal communication). To date, however, the primary function(s) of cardiac AMPK are unclear. We speculate that the primary function of AMPK is to regulate cardiac ACC activity. In recent experiments we observed that AMPK activity is increased in hearts from insulin-resistant rat hearts, which is accompanied by a decrease in ACC activity (Table 10.2).

Based on the data shown in Table 10.2 we hypothesize that activation of AMPK may be a key factor responsible for increased fatty acid oxidation in diabetic rat hearts. Activation of AMPK inhibits ACC, resulting in a decreased production of malonyl CoA, thereby resulting in an increase in fatty acid oxidation. A proposed role of AMPK is shown in Figure 10.1.

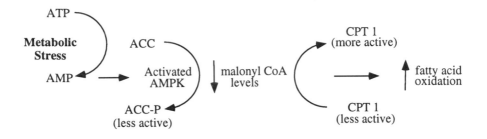

Figure 10.1: **Proposed pathway be which AMP activated protein kinase, Acetyl CoA carboxylase and fatty acid oxidation interact in the diabetic rat heart.** *In diabetes, the activity of AMPK is increased (possibly due to an activation of the kinase that phosphorylates AMPK) resulting in a phosphorylation and inhibition of ACC. Malonyl CoA levels decrease, resulting in a greater activity of CPT 1. Since CPT 1 is critical for mitochondrial fatty acid uptake, fatty acid oxidation are high in the diabetic heart, with a parallel decrease in carbohydrate oxidation.*

To date, little is known about AMPK regulation in the heart. However, the role of AMPK as an inhibitor of liver ACC has recently received considerable attention [79,96,97]. This kinase is allosterically activated by 5'AMP and is activated in situations of cellular stress, such as ATP depletion. In addition to ACC,

AMPK also inactivates hydroxymethylglutaryl (HMG)-CoA reductase [99] and hormone-sensitive lipase [96]. Evidence has suggested that AMPK inhibition by insulin and AMPK stimulation by glucagon can explain the effects of these hormones on ACC [100]. Carling *et al.* [100] recently reported the nucleotide sequence of the catalytic subunit of AMPK, which codes for a 62 kDa protein. AMPK also contains two regulatory subunits which have also recently been cloned by Dr. L. Witters (personal communication). These regulatory subunits contain phosphorylation sites on which another kinase acts to activate AMPK. The allosteric effects of 5'AMP and the promotion of phosphorylation appear to be due to binding of 5'AMP to a single site on the kinase [96,101]. Phosphatase 1C and 2A are capable of reversing the phosphorylation inhibition of AMPK [101].

In support of this proposed model of AMPK in regulating ACC (Figure 10.1), we recently also found that treating cytoplasmic extracts of heart ACC with protein phosphatase 1C will activate the enzyme, providing indirect evidence that heart ACC may be under phosphorylation control.

ß-oxidation of fatty acids and tricarboxylic acid cycle activity

Once in the mitochondrial matrix long-chain acyl-CoA passes through the ß-oxidation enzyme system to produce acetyl-CoA. Each successive cycle of the ß-oxidation spiral results in a 2 carbon shortening of the fatty acid and formation of 1 NADH and 1 $FADH_2$. As mentioned earlier (Table10.1), flux of fatty acids through the ß-oxidation pathway is not impaired and may actually be accelerated in the diabetic rat heart. Direct measurement of the activity of enzymes involved in ß-oxidation support this conclusion. The activity of ß-hydroxyacyl-CoA dehydrogenase (a key enzyme of ß-oxidation) has been shown to be normal [45] or high [102] in diabetic rat mitochondria. The combination of high circulating levels of fatty acids, a decreased regulation of fatty acid uptake by the mitochondria and a normal or accelerated ß-oxidative pathway results in a large proportion of acetyl CoA for the tricarboxylic acid (TCA) cycle being derived from fatty acid oxidation. The accumulation of acetyl-CoA and reduced equivalents from fatty acid ß-oxidation also can dramatically inhibit the pyruvate dehydrogenase complex.

Following the production of acetyl-CoA, the pathways for fatty acid oxidation and glucose oxidation merge. Acetyl-CoA derived from both ß-oxidation and pyruvate dehydrogenase complex (PDHc) enters the TCA cycle, resulting in the liberation of 2 CO_2, 3 NADH and 1 $FADH_2$. Myocardial TCA cycle does not appear to be altered in diabetes. If overall TCA cycle CO_2 production from glucose oxidation and both exogenous and endogenous fatty acid oxidation is measured, no difference in rates are observed in diabetic versus control rats [107]. Measurement of TCA cycle enzyme activities also do not differ in diabetic rats. Furthermore, both citrate synthase and succinate dehydrogenase activities are not altered in diabetic rat hearts [45,102]. As a result, the primary change that occurs in diabetic hearts is not a change in TCA cycle activity, but rather the source of acetyl CoA for the TCA cycle.

Oxidative phosphorylation and ATP synthesis

The next step in ATP production is the entry of NADH derived from glycolysis, the PDHc, the TCA cycle, and ß-oxidation, as well as $FADH_2$ from the TCA cycle and ß-oxidation, into electron transport chain. During passage down the electron transport chain, the hydrogen on NADH and $FADH_2$ is transferred to H_2O in the presence of O_2, and ADP is converted to ATP. Biochemical evidence to date suggests that this process may be impaired in the diabetic. Isolated mitochondrial studies have demonstrated that state 3 respiration and oxidative phosphorylation rates are depressed in the diabetic heart [104-107]. How these alterations in mitochondrial function relate to overall ATP production in the intact heart is still not clear. Although respiration has been shown to be depressed in diabetic heart mitochondria, overall ATP production in the intact heart does not appear to be depressed [9,28]. Rather, the main difference in mitochondrial metabolism appears to be a shift in the source of acetyl CoA for TCA cycle activity. Whether the capacity of mitochondria to produce adequate ATP is compromised at high workloads remains to be determined.

Role of carnitine in fatty acid oxidation

A number of studies have shown that L-carnitine levels are decreased in hearts from diabetic animals [108-112]. This deficiency has been linked to the development of diabetic cardio-myopathies [113]. This is supported by studies demonstrating that L-carnitine treatment is beneficial in improving heart function in experimental diabetes [114-116]. L-Carnitine can also protect the heart in several experimental models of ischemia involving swine, dog, and rat [114-116]. The mechanism(s) responsible for the beneficial effects of L-carnitine are not fully understood, but are generally believed to be related to its actions in reducing myocardial levels of long chain acyl CoA, secondary to a stimulation in fatty acid oxidation. This would restore the long chain acyl CoA to CoA ratio, and subsequently remove the long chain acyl CoA-mediated inhibition of the adenine nucleotide translocase located on the inner mitochondrial membrane [50]. However, a close correlation between long chain acyl CoA levels and heart function has not always been found [117,118]. Furthermore, the popularly held view of L-carnitine action is not consistent with its beneficial effect on the diabetic rat heart, since the heart is already over-reliant on fatty acid oxidation.

In non-diabetic rat hearts L-carnitine can directly stimulate glucose oxidation in the heart [119,120] secondary to an increase in PDHc activity occurring as the result of a decrease the intramitochondrial acetyl CoA/CoA ratio [121]. In fact, in hearts perfused with high levels of fatty acids, addition of L-carnitine actually decreases fatty acid oxidation in parallel with the stimulation of glucose oxidation [119]. Our studies have also suggested that the benefits of L-carnitine in ischemic hearts can be explained by L-carnitine stimulation of glucose oxidation during reperfusion [121]. Recently we demonstrated that L-carnitine can increase glucose oxidation during reperfusion in diabetic rat hearts, and that this is accompanied by an enhanced recovery of mechanical function [122]. This suggests that the beneficial effects of L-carnitine in ischemic hearts from diabetic rats can be explained by overcoming fatty acid inhibition of glucose metabolism.

Endogenous triacylglycerol as a source of fatty acids

Acyl groups present on long-chain acyl-CoA can either be targeted for the mitochondria or incorporated in myocardial triacylglycerol stores. We and others have demonstrated the importance of this endogenous triacylglycerol pool as a source of fatty acids for oxidative metabolism [5,82,123-126]. In the absence of added exogenous fatty acids, isolated working hearts from non-diabetic rats, readily use endogenous triacylglycerol reserves of fatty acids. More than 50% of energy requirements can be met by this source. As increasing concentrations of fatty acids are delivered to the heart, the contribution of these pools to myocardial oxidative metabolism decreases, mainly due to an inhibition of lipolysis. For example, perfusion of isolated working rat hearts with 0.4 mM palmitate and 11 mM glucose results in exogenous fatty acid oxidation rates of 361 ± 68 µmol/g dry wt/min, compared to endogenous triacylglycerol fatty acid oxidation rates of 88.2 ± 13.6 µmol/g wt·min [5]. Even in the presence of high concentrations of fatty acids, however, triacylglycerol fatty acids can account for 11% of total myocardial ATP production [5]. This is achieved due to a rapid turnover of the pool, and suggests myocardial triacylglycerols are a readily mobilizable extended substrate source. We believe, however, that the primary role of triacylglycerol turnover in the aerobic heart is to ensure an adequate supply of fatty acids for ß-oxidation when extracellular fatty acid levels are low.

Diabetes can cause a dramatic increase in myocardial triacylglycerol content [127-129]. These high myocardial triacylglycerol levels are in part related to the high concentrations of plasma free fatty acids [128, 130] and elevated myocardial CoA levels [32] seen in diabetes. We recently determined the relative contribution of this pool to overall myocardial energy require-ments, as well as the relationship between endogenous and exogenous fatty acid oxidation, glycolysis, and glucose oxidation in hearts from streptozotocin diabetic animals. We found that myocardial triacylglycerols can be rapidly mobilized in diabetic rats. In hearts perfused under similar perfusion conditions, triacylglycerol synthesis was not accelerated in diabetic rat hearts compared to control hearts. However, in both the absence and presence of a high concentration of exogenous fatty acid, triacylglycerol lipolysis was significantly enhanced in diabetic rat hearts. In the absence of fatty acids, oxidation of endogenous triacylglycerol fatty acid accounted for 70% of overall myocardial ATP requirements (Figure 10.2). At high levels of fatty acids (1.2 mM palmitate) endogenous triacylglyerol still provided over 10% of the ATP requirements of the heart. Under these conditions, glucose oxidation was essentially abolished.

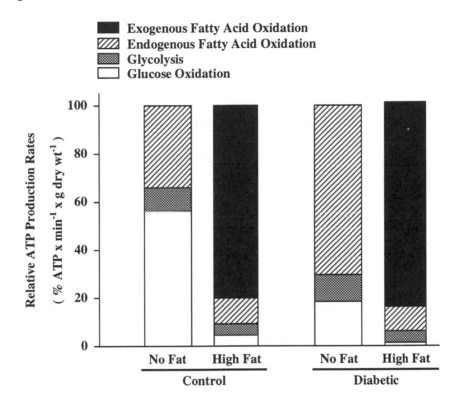

Figure 10.2: Relative contribution of fatty acids and glucose to ATP production in diabetic rat hearts. Rates of ATP production were obtained from isolated working hearts from control and streptozotocin diabetic rats Exogenous and endogenous fatty acid oxidation was performed as previously described [5,28]. By measuring glucose utilization (both glycolysis and glucose oxidation) in a parallel series of hearts perfused under similar conditions we were able to determine the contribution of endogenous triacylglycerol to overall myocardial ATP production. This contribution was determined both in the presence and absence of a high concentration of exogenous fatty acid. Hearts were perfused with Krebs'-Henseleit buffer containing 11 mM glucose, 3% albumin, ±1.2 mM palmitate.

229

Even if diabetic rat hearts are perfused in the absence of fatty acids, glucose oxidation provides less then 20% of the hearts ATP requirements (Figure 10.2). This confirms that high levels of circulating fatty acids are not completely responsible for the decrease in glucose metabolism in diabetic rat hearts. It also supports our hypothesis that regulation of fatty acid oxidation (presumably at the level of malonyl CoA production by ACC) is down regulated in the diabetic heart. This allows for the expanded myocardial triacylglycerol stores seen in diabetic rat hearts to be rapidly mobilized, and provide an alternate source of fatty acids for mitochondrial ß-oxidation in hearts.

Contribution of alterations in fatty acid metabolism to contractile function in the diabetic heart

It has been recognized for many years that diabetics have a significantly greater incidence and severity of angina, acute myocardial infarction (AMI), congestive heart failure, and other manifestations of atherosclerosis compared to the non-diabetic population [131-135]. More recently, it has been determined that ventricular performance can be impaired (diabetic cardiomyopathies) even in the absence of ischemic heart disease [136-144]. Although an increased incidence of atherosclerosis in diabetics contributes to these complications, population-based studies have shown that non-coronary factors are also important contributing factors [145]. For instance, the incidence and severity of complications associated with AMI are greater in the diabetic population even though the size of the infarct is not significantly different, and may even be smaller, compared to the non-diabetic population [146-147]. Diabetes-induced changes within the heart appear to be important contributing factors to injury during and following an AMI [148-150]. Both heart failure following an AMI and diabetic cardiomyopathies have been correlated with the acute metabolic status of the patient [148,151,152]. Furthermore, cardiomyopathies in the absence of ischemic heart disease can be improved by correction of hyperglycemia [153]. Accumulating evidence has implicated changes in myocardial energy substrate use as contributing to diabetic cardiomyopathies [154-160].

Animal studies have confirmed that diabetes-induced changes within the heart are important determinants of diabetic cardio-myopathies and the severity of ischemic injury [135, 136, 161-163]. Biochemical changes that occur within the heart of diabetic animals have been well characterized and include: i) increased collagen content which increases myocardial stiffness, ii) changes in contractile protein function, iii) changes in sarcolemmal and sarcoplasmic reticulum membrane function, iv) changes in mitochondrial function, v) altered characteristics of many of the signal transduction pathways, and vi) changes in the phospholipid membrane characteristics [135-136,157,161-163, also see Chapters 3, 5 and 6]. A large number of studies have shown that preventing one or more of these biochemical changes can improve diabetic heart function [see refs. 150,158,159,161,163 for reviews]. However, despite these promising results, the underlying mechanisms responsible for these changes are still not clear. As will be discussed in the next section, optimizing energy metabolism (both acutely and chronically) will also improve cardiac function in the diabetic heart.

Modification of fatty acid oxidation in the diabetic heart

Previous studies have suggested that fatty acid inhibition of myocardial glucose metabolism is an important contributing factor to the development of both diabetic cardiomyopathies and the increased sensitivity to myocardial ischemic injury [164-167]. These studies have also shown a link between improving glucose utilization and overcoming the biochemical changes that occur in diabetes [168-173]. As a result, interventions aimed at increasing myocardial glucose use should lessen the incidence and severity of these complications.

A number of different pharmacological agents have been shown to acutely improve myocardial performance of isolated hearts obtained from diabetic rats [9,51,122,174]. Both inhibition of fatty acid oxidation [51] or stimulation of glucose oxidation [122,174] results in an improvement of diabetic rat heart function. Chronic interventions that lessen the reliance of the heart on fatty acid oxidation also appear to improve cardiac function in the diabetic rat. These interventions can include direct modification of energy metabolism in the heart, or interventions which modify the supply of fatty acids. Table 10.3 demonstrates that treatment of diabetic rats with a variety of different pharmacological agents can improve

Table 10.3: Interventions which modify lipid levels and heart function in the diabetic rat heart

Intervention	Plasma triacylglycerol	Heart Function	Ref.
Pharmacological			
-CPT-1 inhibitors (POCA, etomoxir methyl palmoxirate oxfenicine)	decreased	improved	168,169 170, 171 172,173 174,175 176
-L-carnitine	decreased	improved	113,177
-myoinositol	decreased	improved	178
-hydralazine	decreased	improved	179,180
-vanadate	decreased	improved	181
-methionine/choline	decreased	improved	182
-T_3	decreased	improved	176
-metformin	decreased	improved	183
Others			
-exercise	decreased	improved	18, 29, 112, 185

myocardial function. Although these agents have diverse pharmacological actions, a common feature is their ability to lower plasma triacylglycerol levels. Whether these agents also lower circulating free fatty acids was not determined in most of these studies. In addition to lowering lipid levels, part of the effects of agents such as CPT-1 inhibitors and carnitine may be related to their direct effect of increasing glucose oxidation in the heart [20,117,119,120,122,165]. Overall, this data supports the concept that high circulating fatty acids and/or a decreased regulation of fatty acid oxidation in the heart contribute to contractile dysfunction.

Summary

In uncontrolled diabetes, hearts have a greater reliance than normal, on fatty acids as fuel. This is due both to high levels of circulating fatty acids and a decreased regulation of fatty acid oxidation in the heart. Pharmacological modification of both circulating lipid levels and the regulation of fatty acid oxidation in the heart can lessen the severity of experimental diabetic cardio-myopathies. The net effect of these interventions is an increase in myocardial glucose metabolism by the heart.

An increase in 5'-AMP activated protein kinase mediated phosphorylation of acetyl CoA carboxylase may be an important mechanism responsible for high fatty acid oxidation rates in the diabetic heart. Inhibition of this kinase and/or activation of acetyl CoA carboxylase may prove to be a useful approach to decrease fatty acid oxidation and increase glucose oxidation in the diabetic heart.

References:

1. Bing RJ. Cardiac metabolism. *Physiol. Rev.* **45**: 171-213, 1964.

2. Goodale WT and Hackel DB. Myocardial carbohydrate metabolism in normal dogs, with effects of hyperglycemia and starvation. *Circ. Res.* **1**: 509-517, 1953.

3. Neely JR and Morgan HE. Relationship between carbohydrate metabolism and energy balance of heart muscle. *Ann. Rev. Physiol.* **36**: 413-459, 1974.

4. Opie LH. Metabolism of the heart in health and disease. *Am. Heart. J.* **76**: 685-689, 1968.

5. Saddik M and Lopaschuk GD. Myocardial triglyceride turnover and contribution to energy substrate utilization in isolated working rat hearts. *J. Biol. Chem.* **266**: 8162-8170, 1991.

6. Garland PB and Randle PJ. Regulation of glucose uptake by muscle. X. Effects of alloxan-diabetes, starvation, hypophysectomy and adrenalectomy and of fatty acids, ketone bodies and pyruvate on the glycerol output and concentrations of free fatty acids, long-chain fatty acyl coenzyme A, glycerol phosphate and citrate cycle intermediates in rat hearts and diaphragm muscles. *Biochem. J.* **93**: 678-687, 1964

7. Randle PJ. Fuel selection in animals. *Biochem. Soc. Trans.* **14**: 799-806, 1986.

8. Goodale WT, Olson RE and Hackel DB. The effects of fasting and diabetes mellitus on myocardial metabolism in man. *Am. J. Med.* **27**: 212-220, 1959.

9. Wall SR and Lopaschuk GD. Glucose oxidation rates in fatty acid-perfused isolated working hearts from diabetic rat. *Biochim. Biophys. Acta* **1006**: 97-103, 1989.

10. Randle PJ, Newsholme EA and Garland PB. Regulation of glucose uptake by muscle: effects of fatty acids, ketone bodies and pyruvate and of alloxan-diabetes and starvation, on the uptake and metabolic fate of glucose in rat heart and diaphragm muscles. *Biochem. J.* **93**: 652-665,

11. Randle PJ, Hales CN, Garland PB and Newsholme EA (1963) The glucose fatty-acid cycle. Its role in insulin sensitivity and the metabolic disturbances of diabetic mellitus. *Lancet* **1**: 785-789, 1963.

12. Newsholme EA, Randle PJ and Manchester KL. Inhibition of the phosphofructokinase reaction in perfused rat hearts by respiration of ketone bodies, fatty acids and pyruvate. *Nature* **193**:270-271, 1962.

13. Kerbey AL, Vary TC and Randle PJ. Molecular mechanism regulating myocardial glucose oxidation. *Basic Res. Cardiol.* **80** (Suppl 2): 93-96, 1985.

14. Randle PJ, Priestman DA, Mistry S and Halsall A. Mechanisms modifying glucose oxidation in diabetes mellitus. *Diabetologia* **37** (Suppl 2): S155-S161, 1994.

15. Reaven GM, Hollenbeck C, Jeng CY, Wu MS and Chen YI. Measurements of plasma glucose, free fatty acid, lactate, and

insulin for 24h in patients with NIDDM. *Diabetes*; **37**: 1020-1024, 1988.

16. Fraze E, Donner CC, Swislocki ALM, Chiou Y-AM, Chen Y-DI and Revean GM. Ambient plasma free fatty acid concentration in noninsulin-dependent diabetes mellitus. *J. Clin. Endocrinol.* **61**: 807-811, 1985.

17. Lopaschuk GD and Spafford MA. Glucose and palmitate oxidation during reperfusion of ischemic hearts from diabetic hearts. *The Diabetic Heart*, Makoto Nagano and Naranjan S. Dhalla Eds. Raven Press 451-464, 1991.

18. Paulson DJ, Mathews R, Bowman J and Zhao J. Metabolic effects of treadmill exercise training on the diabetic heart. *J. Appl. Physiol.* **73**: 265-271, 1992.

19. Chatham JC and Forder JR. A ^{13}C-NMR study of glucose oxidation in the intact functioning rat heart following diabetes-induced cardiomyopathy. *J Mol Cell Cardiol* **25**: 1202-1213, 1993.

20. Broderick TL, Quinney HA and Lopaschuk GD. L-carnitine increase glucose metabolism and mechanical function following ischaemia in the diabetic rat heart. *Cardiovasc. Res.* **25**: 373-378, 1995.

21. Shipp JC. Interelation between carbohydrate and fatty acid metabolism of isolated perfused rat heart. *Metabolism* **13**: 852-867, 1964.

22. Wisnecki JA, Gertz EW, Neese RA and Mayr M. Myocardial metabolism of free fatty acids. *J. Clin. Invest.* **79**: 359-366, 1990.

23. Groop LC, Bonadonna RC, DelPrato S, Ratheiser K, Zyck K, Ferrannini E and DeFronz RA. Glucose and free fatty acid metabolism in non-insulin-dependent diabetes mellitus: evidence for multiple sites of insulin resistance. *J. Clin. Invest.* **84**: 205-213, 1989.

24. Morgan HE, Cadenas E, Regan DM and Park CR. Regulation of glucose uptake in muscle. III. Rate-limiting step and effects of insulin and anoxia in heart muscle from diabetic rats. *J. Biol. Chem.* **236**: 262-268, 1961.

25. Ballard FB, Danforth WH, Naegle S and Bing RJ. Myocardial metabolism of fatty acids. *J. Clin. Invest.* **39**: 717-723, 1960.

26. Evans JR and Hollenberg CH. Lipid metabolism in the diabetic rat heart. *J. Clin. Invest.* **43**: 1234, 1964.

27. Kreisberg RA. Effects of diabetes and starvation on myocardial triglyceride and free fatty acid utilization. *Am. J. Physiol.* **210**: 379-384, 1966.

28. Saddik M and Lopaschuk GD. Triacylglycerol turnover in isolated working hearts of acutely diabetic rats. *Can J Physiol Pharmacol* **72**: 1110-1119, 1994.

29. Paulson DJ, Mathews, Bowman J and Zhao J. Metabolic effects of treadmill exercise training on the diabetic heart. *J. Appl. Physiol.* **73**: 265-271, 1992.

30. Gamble J and Lopaschuk GD. Relationship between fatty acid oxidation and acetyl CoA carboxylase in islet transplanted streptozotocin diabetic rats (Submitted).

31. Lopaschuk GD, Lakey JRT, Barr R, Wambolt R, Thomson ABR, Clandinin MT and Rajotte RV. Islet tranplantation improves glucose oxidation and mechanical function in diabetic rat hearts. *Can. J. Physiol. Pharmacol.* **71**: 896-903, 1993.

32. Lopaschuk GD and Tsang H Metabolism of palmitate in isolated working hearts from spontaneously diabetic "BB" Wistar rats. *Circ. Res.* **61**: 853-858, 1987.

33. Broderick TL, Quinney HA and Lopaschuk GD. Acute insulin withdrawal from diabetic BB rats decreases myocardial glycolysis during low-flow ischemia. *Metabolism* **41**: 332-338, 1992.

34. Lopaschuk GD and Russell JC. Myocardial function and energy substrate metabolism in the insulin-resistant JCR:LA corpulant rat. *J. Appl. Physiol.* **71**: 1302-1308, 1991.

35. Gamble J, Russell JR and Lopaschuk GD. Acetyl CoA carboxylase regulation of atty acid oxidation in hearts of insulin-resistant JCR/LA corpulent rats (Submitted).

36. Howard BV. Lipoprotein metabolism in diabetes mellitus. *J Lipid Res.* **28**: 613, 1987.

37. Nakai T, Oida K, Tamai T, Yamada S, Kobayashi T, Kutsumi Y and Takeda R. Lipoprotein lipase activities in heart muscle of streptoztotocin-induced diabetic rats. *Horm. Metabol. Res.* **16**: 67-70, 1984.

38. Nomura T, Hagino Y, Gotoh M and Iguchi A. The effects of streptozotocin diabetes on tissue specific lipase activities in the rat. *Lipids* **19**: 594-598, 1984.

39. Rodrigues B, Braun JE, Spooner M and Severson DL. Regulation of lipoprotein lipase activity in cardiac myocytes from control and diabetic rat hearts by plasma lipids. *Can. J. Physiol. Pharmacol.* **70**: 1271-1279, 1992.

40. Rodrigues B and Severson DL. Acute diabetes does not reduce heparin-releasable lipoprotein lipase activity in perfused hearts from Wistar-Hyoto rats. *Can. J. Physiol. Pharmacol.* **71**: 657-661, 1993.

41. Braun JE and Severson DL. Diabetes reduces heparin- and phospholipase C-releasable lipoprotein lipase from cardiomyocytes. *Am. J. Physiol.* **260**: E477-E485, 1991.

42. Van der Vusse GJ, Glaztz JFC, Stam HCG and Reneman RS. Fatty acid homeostasis in the normoxic and ischemic heart. *Physiol. Rev.* **72**: 881-940, 1992.

43. Vork MM, Glatz JFC, Surtel DAM, Knubben HJM and Van der Vusse GJ. An enzyme linked immuno-sorben assay for the determination of rat heart fatty acid-binding protein using the streptavidin-biotin system. Application to tissue and effluent samples from normoxic rat heart perfusion. *Biochim. Biophys. Acta* **1075**: 199-205, 1991.

44. Glatz JFC and Van der Vusse GJ. Intracellular faty acid-binding proteins: current concepts and future directions. *Mol. Cell. Biochem.* **98**: 247-251, 1990.

45. Glatz JFC, van Breda E, Keizer HA, de Jong YF, Lakey JRT, Rajotte RV, Thomson A, van der Vusse GJ and Lopaschuk GD. Rat heart fatty acid-binding protein content is increased in experimental diabetes. *Biochem. Biophys. Res. Commun.* **199**: 639-646, 1994.

46. Waku K. Origins and fates of fatty acyl-CoA esters. *Biochim. Biophys. Acta* **1124**: 101-111, 1992.

47. Knudsen J, Mandrup S, Rasmussen JT, Andreasen PH, Poulsen F and Kristiansen K. The function of acyl-CoA binding protein (ACBP)/diazepam binding inhibitor (DBI). *Mol. Cell. Biochem.* **123**: 129-138, 1993.

48. Norman PT, Norseth J, and Thomassen MS. Acyl-CoA synthetase activity of rat heart mitochondria. Substrate specificity with special reference to very-long-chain and isomeric fatty acids. *Biochim. Biophys. Acta* **752**: 474-481, 1983.

49. Corr PB, Gross RW and Sobel BE. Amphipathic metabolites and membrane dysfunction in ischemic myocardium. *Circ. Res.* **55**: 135-154, 1984.

50. Shug AAL, Lerner E, Elson C and Shrago E. Inhibition of adenine nucleotide translocase activity by oleoyl-CoA and its reversal in rat liver mitochondria. *Biochem. Biophys. Res. Commun.* **43**: 557-563, 1971.

51. Pieper GM, Murray WJ, Salhany JM, Wu ST and Elio RS. Salient effects of L-carnitine on adenine-nucloetide loss and coenzyme A acylation in the diabetic heat perfused with excess palmitic acid. *Biochim. Biophys. Acta* **803**: 241-249, 1984.

52. Murthy MSR and Pande SV. Malonyl-CoA binding site and the overt carnitine palmitoyltransferase activity reside on the opposite sides of the outer mitochondrial membrane. *Proc. Natl. Acad. Sci. USA* **84**: 378-382, 1987.

53. Murthy MSR and Pande S. Characterization of a solubilized malonyl-CoA-sensitive CPTase of the inner membrane *Biochem. J.* **84**: 378-382, 1987.

54. Parvin R and Pande SVJ. Enhancement of mitochondrial carnitine and carnitine acylcarnitine transloacase-mediated tarnsport of fatty acids into liver motochondria under ketogenic conditions. *J. Biol. Chem.* **254**: 5423-5429, 1979.

55. Murthy MSR and Pande SV. Some differences in the properties of carnitine palmitoyltransferase activities of the

mitochondrial outer and inner membranes. *Biochem. J.* **248**: 727-733, 1987.

56. Lysiak W, Toth PP, Suelter CH and Bieber LL. Quantification of the efflux of acylcarnitine from rat heart, brain and liver mitochondria. *J. Biol. Chem.* **263**: 13698-13703, 1986.

57. Oram JF, Bennetch SL and Neely JR. Regulation of fatty acid utilization in isolated perfused rat hearts. *J. Biol. Chem.* **2148**: 5299-5309, 1973.

58. McGarry JD, Woeltje KF, Kuwajima M and Foster DW. Regulation of ketogenesis and the renaissance of carnitine palmitoyltransferase. *Diabetes* **5**: 271-284, 1989.

59. McGarry JD, Leatherman GF and Foster DW. Carnitine palmitoyltransferase I. The site of inhibition of hepatic fatty acid oxidation by malonyl-CoA. *J. Biol. Chem.* **253**: 4128-4136, 1978

60. McGarry JD, Mills SE, Long CS and Foster DW. Observations on the affinity for carnitine, and malonyl-CoA sensivity, of carnitine palmitoyltransferase I in animal and human tissues. *Biochem. J.* **214**: 21-28, 1983.

61. Chung CH, Woldegiorgis G, Dai G, Shrago E and Bieber LL. Conferral of malonyl coenzyme A sensitivity to purified rat heart mitochondrial carnitine palmitoyltransferase. *Biochemistry* **31**: 9777-9783, 1992.

62. Ghadiminejad I and Saggerson ED. Carnitine palmitoyl-transferase (CPT2) from liver mitochondrial inner membrane becomes inhibitable by malonyl-CA if reconstituted with outer membrane malonyl-CoA binding protein. *FEBS Lett.* **269**: 406-408, 1990.

63. Cook GA and Gamble MS. Regulation of carnitine palmitoyltransferase by insulin results in decreased activity and decreased apparent K_i values for malonyl CoA. *J. Biol. Chem.* **262**: 2050-2055, 1987.

64. Esser V, Kuwajima M, Britton CH, Krishnan K, Foster DW and McGarry JD. Inibitors of mitochondrial carnitine palmitoyltransferase I limit the action of proteases on the enzyme. *J. Biol. Chem.* **268**: 5810-5816, 1993.

65. Kerner J, Zaluzec E, Gage D and Bieber LL. Characterization of the malonyl-CoA-sensitive carnitine palmitoyltransferase (CPT) of a rat heart mitochondrial particle. *J. Biol. Chem.* **269**: 8209-8219, 1994.

66. McGarry JD and Foster DW. Regulation of hepatic fatty acid oxidation and ketone body production. *Ann. Rev. Biochem.* **49**: 395-420, 1980.

67. Esser V, Britton CH, Weis BC, Foster DW and McGarry JD. Cloning, sequencing, and expression of a cDNA encoding rat liver carnitine palmitoyltransferase I. *J. Biol. Chem.* **268**: 5817-5822, 1993.

68. Weis BC, Esser V, Foster DW and McGarry JD. Rat heart expresses two forms of mitochondrial carnitine palmitoyl-transferase I. *J. Biol. Chem.* **269**: 18712-18715, 1994.

69. Bremer J. The effect of fasting on the activity of liver carnitine palmitoyltransferase and its inhibition by malonyl CoA. *Biochim. Biophys. Acta* **665**: 628-631, 1981.

70. Girard J, Ferre P, Pegorier JP and Duee PH. Adaptations of glucose and fatty aid metabolism during perinatal period and suckling-weaning transition. *Physiol. Rev.* **72**: 507-562, 1992.

71. Saggerson ED and Carpenter CA. Effects of fasting, adrenalectomy and streptozotocin diabetes on snesitivity of hepatic carnitine acyltransferase to malonyl CoA. *FEBS Lett.* **129**: 225-228, 1981.

72. Cook GA and Gamble MS. Regulation of carnitine palmitoyltransferase by insulin results in decreased activity and decreased apparent K_i values for malonyl CoA. *J. Biol. Chem.* **262**: 2050-2055, 1987.

73. Chung CH, Woldegiorgis G, Dai G, Shrago E and Bieber LL. Conferral of malonyl coenzyme A sensitivity to purified rat heart mitochondrial carnitine palmitoyltransferase. *Biochemistry* **31**: 9777-9783, 1992.

74. Cook GA and Lappi MD. Carnitine palmitoyltransferase in the heart is controlled by a different mechanism than the hepatic enzyme. *Mol. Cell. Biochem.* **116**: 39-45, 1992.

75. Lopaschuk GD, Witters LA, Itoi T, Barr R and Barr A. Acetyl CoA carboxylase involvement in the rapid maturation of fatty acid oxidation in the newborn rabbit heart. *J. Biol. Chem.* **269**: 25871-25878, 1994

76. Kudo N, Barr AJ, Barr RL, Desai S and Lopaschuk GD. High rates of fatty acid oxidation during reperfusion of ischemic hearts are associated with a decrease in malonyl-CoA levels due to an increase in 5'-AMP activated protein kinase inhibition of acetyl CoA carboxylase *J. Biol. Chem.* **270**: 17513-17520.

77. Goodridge, AG. Fatty acid synthesis in eucaryotes. In: *Biochemistry of lipids, lipoproteins and membranes.* Vance DE, Vance, J. (eds) 111-139, 1991.

78. Hardie DG. Regulation of fatty acid synthesis via phosphorylation of acetyl CoA-carboxylase. *Prog. Lipid. Res.* **28**: 117-146, 1989.

79. Kim KH, Lopez-Casillas F, Bai DH, Luo X and Pape ME. Role of reversible phosphorylation of acetyl-CoA carboxylase in long-chain fatty acid synthesis. *FASEB* **3**: 2250-2256, 1989.

80. Bianchi A, Evans JL, Iverson AJ, Nordlund A, Watts TD and Witters LA Identification of an isozymic form of acetyl-CoA carboxylase. *J. Biol. Chem.* **265**: 1502-1509, 1990.

81. Hardie DG. Regulation of fatty acid and cholesterol metabolism by the AMP-activated protein kinase. *Biochim. Biophys. Acta* **1123**: 231-238, 1992.

82. Saddik M. Gamble J, Witters LA and Lopaschuk GD. Acetyl-CoA carboxylase regulation of fatty acid oxidation in the heart. *J. Biol. Chem.* **268**: 25836-25845, 1993.

83. Lopaschuk GD, Belke DB, Gamble J, Itoi I and Schönekess BO. Regulation of fatty acid oxidation in the heart. *Biochim. Biophys. Acta* **1213**: 263-276, 1994.

84. Lopaschuk GD and Gamble J. Acetyl-CoA carboxylase: An important regulator of fatty acid oxidation in the heart. *Can. J. Physiol. Pharmacol.* **72**, 1101-1109, 1994.

85. Gamble J, Makinde O and Lopaschuk GD. Acetyl CoA carboxylase activity and expression in the diabetic rat heart (Submitted).

86. Awan MM and Saggerson ED. Malonyl-CoA metabolism in cardiac myocytes and its relevance to the control of fatty acid oxidation. *Biochem. J.* **295**: 61-66, 1993

87. Brun T, Roche E, Kim K and Prentki M. Glucose regulates acetyl-CoA carboxylase gene expression in a pancreatic ß-cell line (INS-1). *J. Biol. Chem.* **268**: 18905-18911, 1993.

88. Prentki M, Vischer S, Glennon MC, Regazzi R, Deeney JT and Coreky BE. Malonyl CoA and long chain acyl-CoA esters as metabolic coupling factors in nutrient-induced insulin secretion. *J. Biol. Chem.* **267**: 5802-5810, 1992.

89. Chen A, Ogawa A, Ohneda M, Unger RH, Foster DW and McGarry JD. More direct evidence for a malonyl CoA-carnitine palmitoyltransferase interaction as a key event in pancreatic ß-cell signalling. *Diabetes* **43**: 887-883, 1994.

90. Kong IS, Lopez-Casillas F and Kim KH. Acetyl-CoA carboxylase mRNA species with or without inhibitory coding sequence for Ser-1200 phosphorylation. *J. Biol. Chem.* **265**:13695-13701, 1990.

91. Lopez-Casillas F and Kim KH. Heterogeneity at the 5' end of rat acetyl-coenzyme A carboxylase mRNA. *J. Biol. Chem.* **264**: 7276-7184, 1989.

92. Lopez-Castillas F, Ponce-Castenada V and Kim KH. Acetyl-Coenzyme A carboxylase mRNA metabolism in the rat liver. *Metabolism* **41**: 201-207, 1992.

93. Louis NA and Witters LA. Glucose regulation of acetyl-CoA carboxylase in hepatoma and islet cells. *J. Biol. Chem.* **267**: 2287-2293, 1992.

94. Mabrouk GM, Helmy IM, Thampy KG and Wakil, SJ. Acute hormonal control of acetyl-CoA carboxylase. *J. Biol. Chem.* **265**: 6330-6338, 1990.

95. Tae H-J, Luo X and Kim K-H. Roles of CCAAT/Enhancer-binding protein and its binding site on repression and derepression of acetyl-CoA carboxylase gene. *J. Biol. Chem.* **269**: 10475-10484, 1994.

96. Hardie DG. Regulation of fatty acid synthesis via phosphorylation of acetyl CoA-carboxylase. *Prog. Lipid Res.* **28**: 117-146, 1989.

97. Hardie DG. Regulation of fatty acid and cholesterol metabolism by the AMP-activated protein kinase. *Biochim. Biophys. Acta* **1123**: 231-238, 1992.

98. Wins R and Hess D, Achersold R and Brownsey RW. Unique structural features and differential phosphorylation of the 280-kDa component (isozyme) of rat liver acetyl-CoA carboxylase. *J. Biol. Chem.* **269**: 14438-14445, 1994.

99. Sato R, Goldstein JL and Brown MS. Replacement of serine-871 of hamster 3-hydroxy-3-methylglutaryl-CoA reductase prevents phosphorylation by AMP-activated kinase and blocks inhibition of sterol synthesis induced by ATP depletion. *Proc. Natl. Acad. Sci. USA* **90**: 9261-9265, 1993.

100. Carling D, Aguan K, Woods A, Verhoeven AJM, Beri RK, Brennan CH, Sidebottom C, Davison D and Scott J. Mammalian AMP-activated protein kinase is homologous to yeast and plant protein kinases involved in the regulation of carbon metabolism. *J. Biol. Chem.* **269**: 11442-11448, 1994.

101. Weekes J, Hawley SA, Corton J, Shugar D and Hardie, D.G. Activation of rat liver AMP-activated protein kinase by kinase kinase in a purified, reconstituted system. *Eur. J. Biochem.* **219**: 751-757, 1994.

102. Chen V, Ianuzzo D, Fong BC and Spitzer JJ. The effects of acute diabetes on myocardial metabolism in rats. *Metabolism* **33**: 1078-1084, 1984.

103. Onishi S, Nunotani H, Fushini H, Tochino Y. k A pathomorphological study on the diabetogenic drug-indueced heart disease in the rat. *J. Mol. Cell. Cardiol.* **13** (Suppl 2): 34, 1982.

104. Savabi F. Mitochondrial creatine phosphkinase deficiency in diabetic rat heart. *Biochem. Biophys. Res. Commun.* **154**: 469-475, 1984.

105. Pierce GN and Dhalla NS. Heart mitochondrial function in chronic experimental diabetes in rats. *Can. J. Cardiol.* **1**: 48-54, 1984.

106. Kuo TH, Moore KH, Giomelli F and Wiener J. Defective oxidative metabolism of heart mitochondria from genetically diabetic mice. *Diabetes* **32**: 781-787, 1983.

107. Mokhtar N, Lavoie J-P, Rousseau-MIgneron S and Nadeau A. Physical training reverses defect in mitochondrial energy production in heart of chronically diabetic rats. *Diabetes* **42**: 686-687, 1993.

108. Feuvray D, Idell-Wenger JA and Neely JR. Effects of ischemia on rat myocardial function and metabolism in diabetes. *Circ Res* **44**: 322-329, 1979.

109. Fogle PJ and Bieber LL. Effect of streptozotocin on carnitine and carnitine acyltransferases in rat heart, liver, and kidney. *Biochem. Med.* **22**: 119-126, 1976.

110. Pearson DJ and Tubbs PK. Carnitine and derivatives in rat tissues. *Biochem. J.* **105**: 953-963, 1967.

111. Vary TC and Neely JR. A mechanism for reduced myocardial carnitine levels in diabetic animals. *Am. J. Physiol.* **243**: H154-H158, 1982.

112. Paulson DJ, Kopp SJ, Peace DG and Tow JP. Myocardial adaptation to endurance exercise training in diabetic rats. *Am. J. Physiol.* **252**: R1073-R1081, 1987.

113. Paulson DJ, Schmidt MJ, Traxler JS, Ramacci MT and Shug AL. Improvement of myocardial function in diabetic rats after treatment with L-carnitine. *Metabolism* **33**: 358-363, 1984.

114. Folts JD, Shug AL, Koke JR and Bittar N. Protection of the ischemic dog myocardium with carnitine. *Am. J. Cardiol.* **41**: 1209-1215, 1978.

115. Liedtke AJ and Nellis SH. Effects of carnitine in ischemic and fatty acid supplemented swine hearts. *J. Clin. Invest.* **64**: 440-447, 1979.

116. Liedtke AJ, Nellis SH, Whitesell LF and Mahar CQ. Metabolic and mechanical effects using L- and D-carnitine in working swine hearts. *Am. J. Physiol.* **243**: H691-H697, 1982.

117. Lopaschuk GD and Spafford M   Response of isolated working hearts from acutely and chronically diabetic rats to fatty acids and carnitine palmitoyltransferase I inhibition during reduction of coronary flow. *Circ Res* **65**: 378-387, 1989.

118. Ichahara K and Nccly JR. Recovery of ventricular function in reperfused ischemic hearts exposed to fatty acids. *Am. J. Physiol.* **249**: H492-H497, 1985.

119. Broderick TL, Quinney H and Lopaschuk GD. Carnitine stimulation of glucose oxidation in the fatty acid perfused isolated working rat heart. *J. Biol. Chem.* **267**: 3758-3763, 1992.

120. Broderick TL, Quinney HA, Barker CC and Lopaschuk GD. The beneficial effect of carnitine on mechanical recovery of rat hearts reperfused after a transient period of global ischemia is accompanied by a stimulation of glucose oxidation. *Circulation* **87**: 972-981, 1994.

121. Lysiak W, Toth PP, Suelter CH and Bieber LL. Quantification of the effect of L-carnitine on the levels of acid-soluble short-chain acyl CoA and CoASH in rat heart and liver mitochondria. *J. Biol. Chem.* **263**: 1511-1156, 1988.

122. Broderick T, Quinney HA and Lopaschuk GD. L-carnitine inreases gluçose metabolism and mechanical function following ischaemia in diabetic rat heart *Cardiovasc. Res.* **29**: 373-378, 1995

123. Saddik M and Lopaschuk GD. Myocardial triglyceride turnover during reperfusion of isolatcd rat hcarts subjcctcd to a transient period of global ischemia. *J. Biol. Chem.* **267**: 3825-3831, 1991.

124. Crass MF. Exogenous substate effects on endogenous lipid metabolism in the working rat hear. *Biochim. Biophys. Acta* **280**: 71-81, 1972.

125 Paulson DJ and Crass MF. Endogenous triacylglycerol metabolism in diabetic heart. *Am. J. Physiol.* **242**: H1084-H1094, 1982.

126 Larsen TS and Severson DL. Influence of exogenous fatty acids and ketone bodies on rates of lipolysis in isolated

ventricular myocytes from normal and diabetic rats. *Can. J. Physiol. Pharmacol.* **68**: 1177-1182, 1990.

127. Denton RM and Randle PJ. Concentration of glycerides and phospholipids in rat heart and gastrocnemius muscles. *Biochem. J.* **104**: 416-422, 1967.

128. Murthy VK and Shipp JC. Accumulation of myocardial triacylglycerols in ketotic diabetes. *Diabetes* **26**: 222-229, 1977.

129. Rizza RA, Crass MF and Shipp JC. Effect of insulin treatment in vivo on heart glycerides and glycogen of alloxan-diabetic rats. *Metabolism* **20**: 539-543, 1974.

130. Murthy VK, Bauman MD and Shipp JC. Regulation of triacylglycerol lipolyiss in the perfused hearts of normal and diabetic rats. *Diabetes* **32**: 718-722, 1983.

131. Bradley RF and Bryfogle JW Survival of diabetic patients after myocardial infarction. *Am. J. Med.* **30**: 207-216, 1956.

132. Kesler I Mortality experience of diabetic patients: a twenty-six year follow-up study. *Am. J. Med.* **51**: 715-724, 1971.

133. Partamian JO and Bradley RF. Acute myocardial infarction in 258 cases of diabetes. *N. Engl. J. Med.* **273**: 455, 1965.

134. Rytter L, Troelsen S and Beck-Nielsen H. Prevalence and mortality of acute myocardial infarction in patients with diabetes. *Diabetes Care* **8**: 230-234, 1985

135. Ulvenstam G, Aberg A, Bergstrand R, Johansson S, Pennert K, Vedin A, Wilhelmsen L and Wilhelmsson C Long-term prognosis after myocardial infarction in men with diabetes. *Diabetes* **34**: 787-792, 1985.

136. Borrow KM, Jaspan JB, Williams KA, Neumann A, Wolinski-Walley P and Lang RM. Myocardial mechanics in young adult patient with diabetes mellitus: Effects of altered load, inotropic state and dynamic exercise. *J. Am. Coll. Cardiol.* **15**: 1508-1517, 1990.

137. Fein FS and Sonnenblick. Diabetic cardiomyopathy. *Prog. Cardiovasc. Dis.* **4**: 255-270, 1985.

138. Hamby RI, Zoneraich and Sherman L. Diabetic cardio-myopathy. *JAMA* **229**: 1749-1754, 1974.

139. Ledet T. Diabetic cardiomyopathy: quantitative histological studies of the heart from young juvenile diabetics. *Acta Path. Microbiol. Scand.* **84**: 421-428, 1976.

140. Mustonen JN, Uusitupa MIJ, Tahvanainen K, Talwar S, Laakso M, Lansimies E, Kuikka JT and Pyorala K. Impaired left ventricular systolic function during exercise in middle-aged insulin-dependent and noninsulin-dependent diabetic subjects without clinically evident cardiovascular disease. *Am. J. Cardiol.* **62**: 1273-1279, 1988.

141. Seneviratne BIB. Diabetic cardiomyopathy: The preclinical phase. *Br. Med. J.* **1**: 1444, 1977.

142. Shapiro LM, Howat AP and Calter MM. Left ventricular function in diabetes mellitus I: Methodology, and prevalence and spectrum of abnormalities. *Br. Heart J.* **45**: 122-128, 1991.

143. Uusitupa M, Mustonen J, Laalso M, Vainio P, Lansimies E, Talwar S and Pyorala K. Impairment of diastolic function in middle-aged Type 1 (insulin-dependent) and Type 2 (non-insulin-dependent) diabetic patients free of cardiovascular disease. *Diabetologia* **31**: 783-791, 1988.

144. Vered,Z, Battler A, Segal P, Liberman D, Yerushalmi Y, Berezin M and Meufeld H. Exercise-induced left ventricular dysfunction in young men with asymptomatic diabetes mellitus (Diabetic cardiomyopathy. *Am. J. Cardiol.* **54**: 633-637, 1984.

145. Kannel WB and McGee DL. Diabetes and cardiovascular risk factors: the Framingham study. *Circulation* **59**: 8-13, 1979.

146. Gwilt DJ, Petri M, Lewis PW, Nattrass M and Pentecost BL Myocardial infarct size and mortality in diabetic patients. *Br. Heart J.* **54**: 466-472, 1985.

147. Harrower AD and Clarke BF. Experience of coronary care in diabetics. *Br. Med. J.* **1**: 126-128, 1976.

148. Jaffe AS, Spadaro JJ, Schechtman K, Roberts R, Geltman EM and Sobel BE Increased congestive heart failure after myocardial infarction of modest extent in patients with diabetes mellitus. *Am. Heart J.* **108**: 31-37, 1984.

149. Stone PH, Muller JE, Hartwel T, York BJ, Rutherford JD, Parker CB, Turi ZG, Strauss HW, Willerson JT, Robertson T, Braunwald E and Jaffe AS. The effect of diabetes mellitus on prognosis and serial left ventricular function after acute myocardial infarction: Contribution of both coronary disease and diastolic left ventricular dysfunction to the adverse prognosis. *J. Am. Coll. Cardiol.* **14**: 49-57, 1989.

150. Götzsche O. Myocardial cell dysfunction in diabetes mellitus. *Diabetes* **35**: 1158-1162, 1986.

151. Oswald B, Corcovan S and Yudkin JS. Prevalence and risks of hyperglycemia and undiagnosed diabetes in patients with acute myocardial infarction. *Lancet* **1**: 1264-1267, 1984.

152. Oswald GA, Smith CCT, Betteridge DJ and Yudkin JS. Determinants and importance of stress hyperglycaemia in non-diabetic patients with myocardial infarction. *Br. Med. J.* **293**: 917-922, 1986.

153. Bellodi G, Manicardi V, Malavasi V, Veneri L, Bernini G, Bossini P, Distefano S, Magnanini G, Muratori L, Rossi G and Zuarini A. Hyperglycemia and prognosis of acute myocardial infarction in patients without diabetes mellitus. *Am. J. Cardiol.* **64**: 885-888, 1989.

154. Miller TB. Cardiac performance of isolated perfused heart from alloxan diabetic rats. *Am. J. Physiol.* **236**: H808-H812, 1972.

155. Penpargkul S, Schaible TF, Yipintsoi T and Scheuer J. The effect of diabetes on performance and metabolism of rat hearts. *Circ. Res.* **47**: 911-921, 1980.

156. Rubler S, Dlugash J, Yuceoglu YZ, Kumral T, Brauwood AW and Grishman AA. A new type of cardiomyopathy associated with diabetic glomerulosclerosis. *Am. J. Cardiol.* **30**: 595-602, 1972.

157. Shapiro LM. Specific heart disease in diabetes mellitus. *Br. Med. J.* **284**: 140-141, 1982.

158. Tahiliani AG and McNeill JH. Diabetes-induced abnormalities in the myocardium. *Life Sci.* **38**: 959-974, 1986.

159. Tomlinson KC, Gardiner SM, Hebden RA and Bennett T. Functional consequences of streptozotocin-induced diabetes

mellitus, with particular reference to the cardiovascular system. *Pharmacol. Rev.* **44**: 103-150, 1992.

160. Paulson DJ, Shug AL, Jurak R and Schmidt M. The role of altered lipid metabolism in the cardiac dysfunction associated with diabetes. In: *The Diabetic Heart* (Ed.: Nagano M, Dhalla NS), pp 395-407, 1991.

161. Dhalla NS, Pierce GN, Innes IR and Beamish RE. Pathogenesis of cardiac dysfunction in diabetes mellitus. *Can. J.Cardiol.* **1**: 263-81, 1985.

162. Kereiakes DJ, Naughton JL, Brudnage B and Schiller NB. The heart in diabetes. *Western J. Med.* **140**: 583-593, 1984.

163. Lopaschuk GD. Alterations in myocardial fatty acid metabolism contribute to ischemic injury in the diabetic. *Can. J. Cardiol.* **5**: 315-320, 1989.

164. Broderick T, Barr RL, Quinney A and Lopaschuk GD. Acute insulin withdrawal from diabetic BB rats decreases myocardial glycolysis during low-flow ischemia. *Metabolism* **41**: 33-338, 1992.

165. Lopaschuk GD, Wall SR, Olley PM and Davies NJ. Etomoxir, a carnitine palmitoyltransferase I inhibitor, protects hearts from fatty acid-induced injury independent of changes in long chain acylcarnitine. *Circ. Res.* **63**: 1036-1043, 1988.

166. Lopaschuk GD, Saddik M, Barr R, Huang L, Barker CC and Muzyka RA. Effects of high levels of fatty acids on functional recovery of ischemic hearts from diabetic rats. *Am. .J Physiol.* **263**: E1046-E1053, 1992.

167. Lopaschuk GD and Spafford M. Acute insulin withdrawal contributes to ischemic heart failure in spontaneously diabetic BB Wistar rats. *Can. J. Physiol. Pharmacol.* **68**: 462-66, 1990.

168. Dillmann WH. Methyl palmoxirate increases Ca^{2+} myosin ATPase activity and changes myosin isoenzyme distribution in the diabetic rat heart. *Am. J. Physiol.* **248**: E602-E605, 1985.

169. Dillmann WH. Myosin isoenzyme distribution and Ca^{2+} activated myosin ATPase activity in the rat heart influenced

by fructose feeding and triiodothyronine. *Endocrinology* **116**: 2160-2166, 1985.

170. Hekimian G and Feuvray D. Reduction of ischemia-induced acyl carnitine accumulation by TDGA and its influence on lactate dehydrogenase release in diabetic rat hearts. *Diabetes* **35**: 906-910, 1986.

171. Rösen P, Herberg L and Reinauer H Different types of posinsulin receptor defects contriubte to insulin resistance in hearts of obese Zucker rats. *Endocrinology* **119**: 1285-1291, 1986.

172. Rupp H, Wahl R and Hansen M. Influence of diet and carnitine palmitoyltransferase I inhibition on myosin and sarcoplasmic reticulum. *J. Appl. Physiol.* **72**: 352-360, 1992.

173. Rösen P and Reinauer H. Inhibition of carnitine palmitoyltransferase 1 by phenylalkyloxiranecarboxylic acid and its influence on lipolyiss and glucose metabolism in isolated, perfused hearts of streptozotocin-daibetic rats *Metabolism* **22**: 177-185, 1984.

174. Nicholl TA, Lopaschuk GD and McNeill JH. Effects of free fatty acids and dichloroacetate on isolated working diabetic rat heart. *Am. J. Physiol.* **261**: 1053-1059, 1991.

175. Collier GR, Traianedes K, Macaulay SL and O'Dea K. Effect of fatty acid oxidation inhibition on glucose metabolism in diabetic rats. *Horm. Metab. Res.* **25**: 9-12, 1993.

176. Foley JF. Rationale and application of fatty acid oxidation inhibitors in treatment of diabetes mellitus. *Diabetes Care* **15**: 773-784, 1993.

177. Tahiliani AG and McNeill JH. Prevention of diabetes-induced myocardial dysfunction in rats by methylpalmoxirate and triiodothryonine treatment. *Can. J. Physiol. Pharmacol.* **63**: 925- 931, 1985.

178. Rodrigues B, Xiang H and McNeill JH. Effect of L-carnitine treatment on lipid metabolism and cardiac performance in chronically diabetic rats. *Diabetes* **37**: 1358-1364, 1988.

179. Xiang H, Heyliger CE and McNeill JH. Effect of myo-inositol and T_3 on myocardial lipiods and cardiac function in streptozotocin diabetc rats. *Diabetes* **37**: 1542-1548, 1988.

180. Burns AH, Racey Burns LA, Jurenka LU and Summer WR. Myocardial metaboalic effects of in vivo hydralazine treatment of streptozotocin-diabetic rats. *Am. J. Physiol.* **260**: H516-H521, 1991.

181. Rodrigues G, Goyal RK and McNeill JH. Effects of hydralazine on streptozotocin-induced diabetic rats: prevention of hyperlipidemia an dimprovement of cardiac function. *J. Pharmacol. Expt. Therap.* **237**: 292-299, 1986.

182. Heyliger CE, Rodriques B and McNeill JH. Effect of choline an methionine treatment on cardiac dysfunction of diabetic rats. *Diabetes* **35**: 1152-1157, 1988.

183. Heyliger CE. Tahiliani AG and McNeill JH. Effect of vanadate on elevated blood glucose and depressed cardiac performance of diabetic rats. *Science* **227**: 1474-1476, 1985.

184. Verma S and McNeill JH. Metformin improves cardiac function in isolated streptozotocin-daibetic rat hearts. *Am. J. Physiol.* **266**: H714-H719, 1994.

185. Tan MH, Bonen A, Garner JB and Belcastro AN. Physical training in diabetic rats: effects on glucose tolerance and serum lipids. *J. Appl. Physiol.* **52**: 1514-1518, 1982.

CHAPTER 11

Conclusion

John C. Chatham
John R. Forder
John H. McNeill

Diabetes mellitus is a major public health problem estimated to affect 80 million people world wide in 1990; this is expected to double by the year 2000 [1]. In the United States alone approximately 12 million people have diabetes [2] and this number is increasing each year [3]. Cardiovascular disease accounts for the majority of the morbidity and mortality in diabetes; in the USA in 1987 over 1 million diabetics were hospitalized with either cardiovascular disease or ischemic heart disease as the primary diagnosis -- more than 100,000 died [3]. It has been shown that following acute myocardial infarction mortality rates were two-fold higher in patients with non-insulin dependent diabetes mellitus (NIDDM) when compared to non-diabetics with similar sized infarcts [4]. Uusitupa *et al.* [5] showed that the age adjusted cardiovascular mortality rates were more than 8 fold higher in diabetics compared to non-diabetic subjects -- principally as a result of an increased incidence of coronary heart disease. Stamler and colleagues also reported that diabetes is an independent risk factor for cardiovascular disease, over and above risk factors such as serum cholesterol, blood pressure and cigarettes [6]. It is also clear that there is a marked incidence of heart failure in diabetic patients that is independent of other risk factors of heart disease, such as hypertension and atherosclerosis [7-9]. Despite the significance of heart disease in limiting the quality and longevity of life for diabetic patients, there is no consensus as to the mechanisms involved or the most appropriate treatment strategies required to minimize these risks.

It is commonly presumed that good metabolic control of diabetics will decrease the risk of cardiovascular disease; however there is little direct evidence to support this conclusion. The recently completed Diabetes Control and Complications Trial showed that intensive insulin therapy had a significant effect on the development of retinopathy, nephropathy and neuropathy, but little data was presented regarding cardiovascular disease [10]. When considering all cardiovascular and peripheral vascular events they found that intensive insulin therapy had no significant effect. However, this study examined relatively young patients (13-39 years), which may preclude the possibility of detecting treatment-related differences. Eschwège et al. [11] reported that there was no relationship between the duration of diabetes or the level of blood glucose and the severity or incidence of coronary heart disease, . In contrast, others have shown that in diabetic subjects in the highest tertile of fasting blood glucose, cardiovascular mortality was three times higher than those in the lowest tertile [5]. This suggests that poor metabolic control may result in an increased risk of cardiovascular disease. There is also some evidence to suggest that treatment with insulin or other hypoglycemic therapy can reverse some of the hemodynamic alterations that are apparent in both insulin dependent diabetes mellitus (IDDM) and NIDDM patients (see Chapter 1 for more details). Experimentally it has been shown that insulin treatment is the single most effective agent in reversing at least some of the detrimental effects of diabetes on the heart (Chapter 4). It has also been shown that agents that are specifically either hypoglycemic (i.e., phlorizin) or hypolipidemic (i.e., hydralazine) are also beneficial.

One of the problems associated with understanding the underlying pathophysiology of diabetes associated heart disease is the wide range of systemic and cardiovascular alterations that occur, many of which are themselves independent risk factors for heart disease (see Table 11.1). In addition, many of the functional and morphological changes that are observed are common to

Table 11.1: Summary of the systemic, functional and morphological alterations to the cardiovascular system during diabetes. These represent the major changes discussed in more detail principally in Chapters 1-3.

Systemic	Functional	Morphologic
Hypoinsulinemia	Increased LVED pressure	Atherosclerosis
Hyperglycemia		Large vessel disease: *Basement membrane thickening*
Hyperlipidemia	Increased wall stiffness	
Ketosis	Reduced ejection fraction	Small vessel disease: *Micro-aneurysms*
Hypertension	Decreased fractional shortening	Fibrosis: *Perivascular, interstitial and replacement*
Increased thrombin production	Decreased rate of LV filling	
Decreased fibrinolysis		LV and RV hypertrophy
Increased platelet activity	Increase in action potential duration	Myocytolysis
		Increased glyco-protein deposition

congestive heart failure of any etiology. Most experimental studies have focused on either STZ- or alloxan-induced diabetes which are most closely related to IDDM; whereas, 90% of patients have (NIDDM). Although both groups of patients have increased incidence of heart disease [5], it is not known whether the etiology is the same.

Following diabetes there are a multitude of alterations to both the myocardium and the vascular system, from the molecular and sub-cellular level through to myocyte loss, fibrosis and impaired contractile function (see Tables 11.1 and 11.2). From both a clinical and experimental point of view perhaps one of the most important questions is -- What is the sequence of events that leads to the cardiac dysfunction that occurs during diabetes? There have been very few investigations that have combined long term studies

Table 11.2: Summary of the effects of diabetes on metabolic/biochemical processes and membrane function in the heart. These represent the major changes that occur at the subcellular level and are discussed in more detail principally in Chapters 5-10. Where known the putative causes for the observed changes are shown in italics.

Metabolic/Biochemical	Membrane function
Decreased glucose transport: *Decrease in GLUT4 expression and GLUT4 mRNA*	Decreased myosin Ca^{2+}-ATPase activity: *Shift from V_1 to V_3 myosin isoform*
Decreased hexokinase activity : *Decrease in hexokinase II expression and mRNA*	Decreased SR Ca^{2+} pump activities: *Accumulation of long-chain acylcarnitines*
Decreased glucose oxidation: *Increased PDH kinase activity resulting in an decrease of PDH in active form*	Decreased mitochondrial calcium uptake
Decreased glycogen synthase	Decreased in number of sarcolemmal Ca^{2+}-channels
Decreased glycogen phosphorylase	Impaired function and decreased number of α- and ß-adrenergic receptors
Increased fatty acid oxidation: *Decreased acetyl-CoA carboxylase activity, due to increased AMP activated protein kinase leading to a reduction in malonyl-CoA*	Decrease in sarcolemmal Na^+-K^+ ATPase and Ca^{2+}-ATPase
Depressed mitochondrial function: *Altered calcium handling*	Decrease in sarcolemmal Na^+-Ca^{2+} exchange
Decreased protein synthesis: *Decrease in translational efficiency*	Decreased sarcolemmal content of phosphatidylethanolamine and diphosphatidylglycerol
Decreased creatine kinase activity: *Decrease in creatine kinase mRNA activity*	

of the effects of diabetes on cardiac function with studies at the subcellular and molecular level. Nevertheless, it is possible to construct a chronology of events that occur following the onset of experimental diabetes. For example, changes in tissue morphology appears to be a relatively late event, while changes at the subcellular and/or molecular level are among some of the earlier changes to take place following the induction of diabetes (See Figure 11.1).

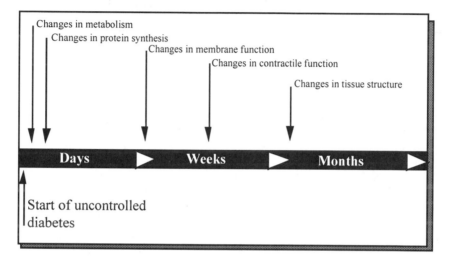

Figure 11.1: Chronology of events that occur in the myocardium following the initiation of uncontrolled experimental diabetes. Clearly there is some variability regarding the precise timing of these events depending on the exact model of diabetes used. It remains to be determined whether, insulin treatment or hypoglycemic therapy prevents completely or simply delays these changes.

Changes in intermediary metabolism appear to precede all other changes in the myocardium induced by diabetes. For example, diabetes leads to decreased myocardial glucose utilization which has been observed as little as 48 hours after the induction of diabetes and becomes progressively worse with the duration of diabetes. Similar results have been observed in both animal models as well as patients (See Chapter 9). This decrease in glucose utilization is accompanied by an increase in fatty acid metabolism (See Chapter 10). It has been suggested that the combination of an inhibition of glucose oxidation combined with stimulation of fatty acid metabolism may make the heart more susceptible to ischemic injury. However, it is unclear whether such changes also increase the risk of heart failure. It is tempting to propose that alterations in intermediary metabolism may be the underlying cause of both the development of diabetic cardiomyopathy as well as the increased susceptibility to ischemic injury; however, much more work is required before a causal relationship is established.

There are a multitude of other subcellular and membrane changes in the myocardium that may also be implicated in the development of diabetic cardiomyopathy, many of which involve alterations in calcium handling (see Chapters 3 and 6). Since calcium is central both to contractile function as well as the regulation of many other metabolic processes, it is possible that changes in calcium handling could play an important role in diabetes induced cardiac dysfunction.

It has been proposed that an increase in collagen deposition results in an increased stiffness of the myocardium, which leads to impaired diastolic function in the diabetic heart (Chapter 3). However, the time course of collagen deposition relative to the development of diastolic dysfunction remains to be determined. An increase in collagen may be an essential step in the development of cardiac dysfunction; although it is also possible that the increase in collagen is secondary to other changes.

Due to the myriad and diverse effects of diabetes on the heart it is unlikely that there is any single factor that precipitates the decline in cardiac performance. Nevertheless, it is possible that the combination of relatively few factors could precipitate the chain of events leading to impaired contractile function and ultimately failure. It is also likely that subtle molecular and biochemical alterations will precede the marked pathophysiological changes that accompany the diabetic cardiomyopathy. Therefore, in order to better understand the evolution of diabetes-induced cardiac injury it is essential for future work not only to delineate the effects of diabetes on the heart, but more importantly to focus on the evolution and interrelationship between the various changes that occur.

References

1. Zimmet P. Diabetes care and prevention - around the world in 80 days. In H Rifkin,JA Colwell and SI Taylor (Eds.), *"Diabetes"* (pp. 721-729). Elsevier, 1991.

2. Lasker RD. The diabetes control and complications trial. Implications for policy and practice. *N. Engl. J. Med.* **329**: 1035-1036, 1993.

3. Wetterhall SF, Olson DR, DeStefano F, Stevenson JM, Ford ES, German RR, Will JC, Newman JM, Sepe SJ and Vinicor F. Trends in diabetes and diabetic complications, 1980-1987. *Diabetes Care* **15**: 960-967, 1992.

4. Lehto S, Pyorala K, Miettinen H, Ronnemaa T, Palomaki P, Tuomilehto J and Laakso M. Myocardial infarct size and mortality in patients with noninsulin-dependent diabetes mellitus. *J Intern Med* **236**: 291-297, 1994.

5. Uusitupa MIJ, Niskanen LK, Siitonen O, Voutilainen E and Pyorala K. 10-Year cardiovascular mortality in relation to risk factors and abnormalities in lipoprotein composition in type-2 (Non-Insulin-Dependent) diabetic and Non-Diabetic subjects. *Diabetologia* **36**: 1175-1184, 1993.

6. Stamler J, Vaccaro O, Neaton JD and Wentworth D. Diabetes, other risk factors, and 12-yr cardiovascular mortality for men screened in the multiple risk factor intervention trial. *Diabetes Care* **16**: 434-444, 1993.

7. Kannel WB, Hjortland M and Castelli WP. Role of diabetes in congestive heart failure: The Framingham Study. *Am. J. Cardiol.* **34**: 29-34, 1974.

8. Kannel WB and McGee DL. Diabetes and cardiovascular risk factors: The Framingham study. *Circulation* **59**: 8-13, 1979.

9. Kannel WB and McGee DL. Diabetes and cardiovascular disease: The Framingham study. *JAMA* **241**: 2035-2038, 1979.

10. The DCCT Research Group: The effect of intensive treatment of diabetes on the development and progression of long-term complications in insulin-dependent diabetes mellitus. *N. Eng. J. Med.* **329**: 977-986, 1993.

11. Eschwège E, Balkau B and Fontbonne A. The epidemiology of coronary heart disease in glucose intolerant and diabetic subjects. *J. Int. Med.* **236** (Suppl.): 5-11, 1994.

INDEX

Acetate 174
acetoacetate 145, 146, 150-153, 175
acetoacetyl-CoA 145-147, 151, 152
acetoacetyl-CoA thiolase 145-147, 149
acetone 145
acetyl-CoA 72, 145, 147, 156, 174 195, 197, 201-203, 225
acetyl-CoA carboxylase (ACC) 221-223, 225, 230, 255
acetylcholine 50, 55
action potential duration 31, 49, 50, 254
actomyosin 69, 75, 93, 101, 103
acyl-CoA synthetase 219, 220
adenine nucleotide translocase 227
adenylate cyclase 69, 115, 176
adrenergic receptors 125
    alpha-receptor 114, 117, 118 168, 171, 255
    beta-receptor 32, 49, 74, 93, 114-118, 168, 171, 177-179, 181, 255
alanine 197, 198
aldose reductase 53
aldose reductase inhibitors 51
alpha-receptors --see adrenergic receptors
amino acids 85-87, 216
aminoacyl transfer RNA (tRNA) 85
anaplerosis 156, 157
angiotensin converting enzyme (ACE) 42
angiotensin II 43, 93
anoxia 166, 171, 177, 180
arachidonic acid 123
arrhythmias 31, 50, 51, 57, 68, 108
arrhythmogenesis 50
ATP synthesis 32, 109, 218, 226
ATPase
    calcium 32, 69, 73, 102-106, 120
        actomyosin 69, 75

        myofibrillar 102, 103, 113, 125
        myosin 44-46, 69, 77, 93, 101, 103-105, 255
        sarcolemma 120, 121, 255
        sarcoplasmic reticulum 107
    magnesium 70, 102, 106, 111
    myosin, potassium-EDTA 103
    sodium-potassium 51-53, 56, 69, 77, 118-121, 123, 126, 255
        p-nitrophenyl phosphatase senstitive 119
atrial conduction 49
atrial filling velocity 12
atrophy 91
autonomic nervous system 50
autonomic neuropathy --see neuropathy

Basement membrane 7, 25, 69, 124
BB/Worcester spontaneously diabetic rats 45, 71, 166, 172, 178, 217
beta-receptors --see adrenergic receptors
bradycardia 46, 114, 117

Caffeine 177
calcium
    channels 111-114, 121, 125, 255
        voltage sensitive, L-type 112, 113
        T-type 111, 112
    channel blocker --see verapamil
    homeostasis 69, 77, 100
    loading 50
    overload 104, 108, 113
    uptake 52
        mitochondria 70, 108, 110, 255

262

phospholipids
    N-methylation 123
    phosphatidyl inositol 52, 53, 57
    phosphatidylcholine 73, 122, 123
    phosphatidylethanolamine 48, 122, 255
phosphocreatine 109, 110, 181
phosphofructokinase 175, 194
phosphoglucomutase 168
positron emission tomography 205
potassium
    current 50, 56
    myocardial content 51, 53, 56, 118
    transport 118
prazosin 75, 179 -- *see also adrenergic receptors, alpha*
propranolol 179 -- *see also adrenergic receptors, beta*
protein degradation
    effect of diabetes 89, 90
    effect of insulin 87, 88
    measurement of 86
    -- *see also protein synthesis*
protein kinases 49, 167, 179
    5'AMP dependent (AMPK) 223, 224, 233, 255
    cAMP dependent 120, 121, 168, 170, 171, 177, 223
    C 118
    calcium dependent 120, 121, 168
    insulin stimulated 169, 170
    -- *see also glycogen phosphorylase kinase and synthase kinase*
protein phosphatases 167-170, 180
    1C 225
    2A 170
    glycogen associated, phosphatase-1 (PP1-G) 169
protein synthesis 32, 49, 85-94, 173, 255
    effect of diabetes 89-92
    effect of fatty acids 89
    effect of insulin 87
    fetal 88

    measurement of 85-87
    -- *see also contractile proteins, synthesis of*
    -- *see also peptide chain initiation and elongation*
protein turnover -- *see protein synthesis and degradation*
proteinuria 12
pseudo-ketogenesis 146
pyruvate 145, 174, 190, 195, 197, 201-205
    efflux 195
    oxidation 150,166, 195, 202
pyruvate dehydrogenase complex (PDHc) 72, 76, 149, 150, 157, 175, 190, 198-201, 207, 215, 226, 227
    kinase 150, 202-204, 207, 215, 255
    kinase activator protein 204
    phosphatase 202

Radionuclide angiocardiography 47
radionuclide ventriculography 13
receptors -- *see adrenergic receptors*
retinopathy 9-15, 27, 253
ribosomes 49
    concentration 89
    content 90, 92
    degradation, 90
    RNA 91
    synthesis 88, 90
    -- *see also protein synthesis*

Sarcolemma 69, 100, 101, 105, 111-124, 191, 219, 231, 255
    calcium binding 32, 124
    calcium uptake -- *see calcium uptake, sarcolemma*
    composition 48, 122-124, permeability 69, 122
    -- *see also ATPase, calcium and membrane*
sarcoplasmic reticulum 32, 45, 48, 52, 69, 75, 77, 100, 101, 104-108, 231 -- *see also calcium uptake, sarcoplasmic reticulum and ATPase, calcium*
selenium 72

silent myocardial ischemia -- *see ischemic heart disease*
small vessel disease 4-7, 11-15, 29-32, 66, 205, 254
sodium
    accumulation 51-53, 57, 119

    -calcium exchange 52, 56, 69, 119, 120, 123
    -proton exchange 52, 121
    selenate -- *see selenium*
    transport 52, 118, 120
    -- see also ATPase, sodium-potassium
sorbitol 53, 54
succinate dehydrogenase 109, 226
sudden death 31, 51
sympathetic nervous system 10, 14, 50-53, 57, 116 -- *see also adrenergic receptor*
systolic function -- *see left ventricular function*

Tachycardia 30, 31
thallium scans 7
thrombin production 26, 254
thyroid hormone 46, 74, ,75, 116
    plasma levels 45, 46, 117
    thyroxine (T_4) 46, 106, 116
    thyroidectomy 116
    thyroiditis 45
    triiodothyronine (T_3) 46, 75, 117
    -- see also hypothyroidism
timolol, 118 -- *see also adrenergic receptors, beta*
tolbutamide 42
triacylglycerol 218, 228
    lipolysis 229
    myocardial content 75, 228, 230
    serum levels 175, 232
    synthesis 228
    turnover 217, 218, 228
tricarboxylic acid (TCA) cycle 144, 146, 151, 197-201, 207, 225, 226
    effect of ketone bodies 153-158
triglycerides 26, 32, 48, 68, 73, 152

    myocardial content 6, 48, 68, 73, 152
    serum levels 73-76, 75,167, 197
    -- see also hypertriglyceridemia and fatty acids
tropomyosin 86, 93
troponin 86, 93, 101

Uridine diphosphate (UDP) 171
uridine diphosphoglucose (UDPG) 167-172
    pyrophosphorylase (UDPG-PP) 168
uridine triphosphate (UTP) 171

Vagal tone 51 -- *see also sympathetic nervous system*
vanadium 70-72, 232
vascular resistance 9, 27
vasospasm 30
verapamil 30, 75, 76, 103, 104, 107, 108, 112, 113 -- *see also calcium channels*